"Thank you for letting us into your lives and sharing your story with the entire country. We have been getting so many calls and comments on how touched people have been by hearing your story." —Francine Weinberg, producer, Pax TV segment *It's a Miracle,* September, 2000

"Gaea Shaw never met Christopher Kuhlman. But she feels that he's very much a part of her. . . . His heart was transplanted into Shaw, a sufferer of genetic heart disease. Barely two months later, Shaw took up competitive swimming and went on to win three medals at the U.S. Transplant Games. Oddly, Kuhlman's passions in life had been skiing and swimming. In a tearful gathering on Valentine's Day, Kuhlman's family met Shaw and her family. Now the Kuhlmans proudly display one of Shaw's medals in their home, a gift from a woman who says she's not sure she can ever adequately express her thanks." —*Denver Rocky Mountain News/Daily Camera,* April 18, 1999

"Swimming became her passion after she received Christopher's heart. Only later did she discover that it had been his passion as well." —Jane Stubbins, *Summit Daily News,* March 14, 1999

"Gaea Shaw's heart was weakening every day, and without a transplant, she wouldn't survive to see her daughter grow up. Then a caring family gave her the gift of life. Now she wondered, what could she do in return?" —Peg Verone, *Woman's World,* July 4, 2000

"Her new heart racing, Gaea Shaw was poised to meet the family who had given her a second chance at life. For Joni and George Kuhlman, the moment was bittersweet—coming face-to-face with the woman who now has their son Christopher's heart. Gaea Shaw and Joni Kuhlman smiled at one another, then embraced and cried. Kuhlman placed her hand over Shaw's heart—the heart that once had beaten for her own son.

'Wow,' she said, choking back tears. 'It's beating really hard.'

'You're so beautiful,' answered Shaw, tears rolling down her face, too. 'It's a wonderful heart. I knew it right away.'" —Carlos Illescas, *The Denver Post*, February 15, 1999

Dying to Live

Dying to Live

From Heart Transplant
to Abundant Life

Gaea Shaw

*From my heart
to yours,
Gaea Shaw*

Dying to Live

From Heart Transplant to Abundant Life

Gaea Shaw

Content © 2005 by Gaea Shaw

Book Design © 2005 by Pilgrims Process, Inc.

Photo credits: Bob Garypie for www.TransWeb.org: All about Transplantation and Donation–cover, p. 61; dona laurita/laurita fotografia–p.43; Colorado Hometown Newspapers 2005, published with permission–p. 58; Sara Shaw–p. 62; Reel Kids–p. 66; *The Denver Post*–pp. 67, 68; Kate Lunz–p. 74

ISBN: 09749597-5-8

Library of Congress Control Number:

2005902059

Printed in the United States of America

0 9 8 7 6 5 4 3 2 1

Typeset in Brush Script Std (various sizes) and Minion Pro (11 pt) using Adobe inDesign CS

To Christopher, who gave life to so many.

To the Kuhlmans and donor families everywhere.

To my husband, Barry—your love and devotion are magnificent.

To my daughter, Sara—you are strong and courageous; I love you forever.

To my beloved sister, Joanne—you are always by my side.

Acknowledgments

This story poured out in a burst of creative energy. Friends and writers who saw the first draft all said the same thing: it showed great potential; it needed rewriting; and I was the one to do it. Thanks to Helene Aarons, Deborah Drier, Elissa Lewis, Paulette Millander, and Pam Novotny for encouraging me to continue working on my manuscript.

My husband, Barry, came home one day with the business card of a local author and writing coach named Susan Griffin. We worked together for many months, through many revisions, until the very last word was in place. I thank Susan for cheering me on, asking all the right questions, and guiding me to a passion for writing. Susan's style was to guide, not to take over. I can proudly say every word in this book is mine. Susan, I am enormously grateful for your brilliant and insightful mentoring.

Thanks to Susan Booker, Jennifer Delaney, and Valerie Monroe, my readers. They offered thoughtful, honest, and direct feedback, and the book is better for it.

My husband, Barry, and daughter, Sara, have been my main support team all along. When writing became my passion and I disappeared behind my office door for hours on end, you never complained or interrupted. Thank you!

This is my first book and the publishing world is new to me. What could have been cold and impersonal melted into warmth and caring with Gary White and Elyn Aviva at Pilgrims Process, Inc.. I am grateful for their guidance, support, expertise, collaborative style, and their reminders that we could have fun with the process.

I always feel gratitude for Christopher, my heart donor. To live life fully in his honor is the only way for me to live.

Contents

Introduction

This book is about facing challenges. Being miserable. Finding faith. Opening up to support. Not being so darned self-sufficient. It chronicles a time in my life that was filled with pain, fear, anger, yearning, learning, love, challenge, hope, trust, and joy.

This is the story of my heart transplant journey, but it is also about so much more. Not everyone faces a heart transplant. But most people face challenges, heartbreak, fear, anger, loneliness, frustration, and adversity in one form or another.

Life can be fulfilling regardless of circumstances. We have choices; we can act. I know that now. I didn't know it on a cool November night in Los Angeles when a five-foot nine, one-hundred-eighty-pound mountain man opened the door at my friend's party.

1983

I met my husband Barry when I was forty-three and he was thirty-seven.

I can picture him now with his strong, clear features, wearing a flannel shirt, jeans, and hiking boots—the epitome of rugged fitness. It was love at first sight for him. For me, it took about ten days. He was moving to Boulder, Colorado, three weeks later, following his heart's desire to be in the mountains, away from the traffic and craziness of the big city. He was starting all over again, with no work in sight, with just the passion to be true to himself. Meeting me complicated things for him because he was afraid I would keep him from achieving his goal. He didn't know that years before we met I promised myself that if the right person showed up in my life, I would follow him anywhere. I was a teacher, after all, and I could always get work. We spent lots of time together before he left, but leave he did.

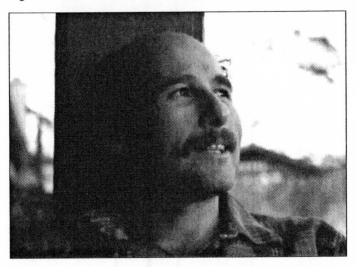

1983, Mountain Man Barry

I was with him when he said goodbye to his mother. They held each other, hugged, and cried. All these years later, as I see the depth of this man's loyalty and love for his family and friends, I realize how much a measure of his character those precious moments with his mother were.

For the next six months, as Barry settled in and found work in Boulder, he sent me three love letters a day and called every night. Six months later I had a teaching job in Boulder and we were married. I married someone I hardly knew. But I was forty-three and figured I had learned something in all those years, so I just went for it.

The wedding took place on June 17, 1984, in his brother and sister-in-law's backyard in Westwood Village, California. We didn't have much money and a fancy wedding wasn't possible, so friends catered the affair. The day was glorious, the food scrumptious, and everyone had a good time. Asking friends to help was out of character for me then. Much later, when I was very sick, asking for help became a lesson about giving and receiving that would be crucial for the rest of my life.

My sister, Joanne, was my matron of honor. Ever since I was very young, I have been devoted to and deeply in love with Joanne. I treasure the photos of her from my wedding day: there she is, petite in stature, with a bit of a moon face, wearing a lovely Indian dress and gauzy hat, being so present and loving with me. Neither of us knew then that we were both genetically coded for big trouble. It was simply a beautiful day.

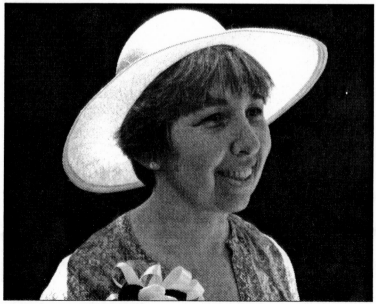

Wedding Day, my sister Joanne

Barry and I honeymooned in San Diego and then drove to Boulder. We arrived in the middle of the night at the house Barry had rented for us. In the next morning's light, standing in the front yard with its one very tall elm tree and its beautiful, extensive lawn, Barry told me that just before he came back to Los Angeles for our wedding he had, on hands and knees, used clippers to cut the entire lawn because he didn't have a lawnmower. I was beginning to learn about the perseverance and fortitude of this new person in my life.

We didn't know then that I had a time bomb ticking in me in the form of an inherited heart disease called cardiomyopathy. In less than ten years it would threaten my life and take my sister's and two cousins' lives. It would cause my cousin Mel to get a heart transplant, and lead me to a heart transplant.

We also didn't know that we would be tested physically, emotionally, and spiritually to face that enormous challenge. During those next ten years, we would discover ways to access our own strength, determination, and faith, as well as to accept support from community, family, and friends. When Barry and I started our life together, however, we knew nothing of what lay ahead.

Barry loved babies and children, so it wasn't long before the topic of parenting surfaced. Many younger couples are advised to discuss this, as well as many other critical relationship topics, before they marry. We just got married and discussed everything afterwards. I wasn't sure I wanted children, but certainly my biological clock was ticking and I didn't have a whole lot of years to consider the issue. I took deeply to heart the advice of my sister. She said that parenting, under the best of circumstances is so challenging that she hoped I'd wait for a completely green light before entering the process.

The green light turned on in the spring of 1986 when we were vacationing at the hot springs in Glenwood Springs, Colorado. Watching families playing in the pool, seeing the joy of that connection, was a big "yes" for me. That decision, like the decision to marry Barry, came from my heart not my head. My beautiful heart was guiding my life, and I was listening. Pregnancy didn't happen, though, and time was passing. We decided to consider adoption, and on March

10, 1988, nine months after our call to an adoption agency, we held Sara Rachael Shaw in our arms for the first time. She was five weeks old and awesomely beautiful, with big blue eyes and light blond peach fuzz for hair. I was a mother and my whole life changed. By that time I was forty-seven years old, five years away from my first hospitalization and nine years away from a heart transplant.

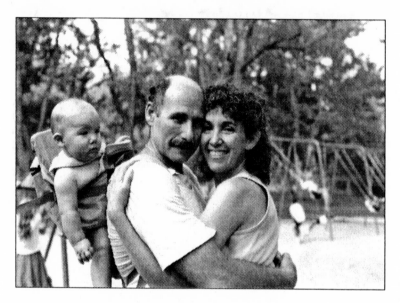

At the park, Sara, Barry, and me

Most people have no idea of what goes on with a person who is waiting for a transplant. Each journey is unique, but one thing is common to everyone on that waiting list. They were living normal and healthy lives before they became ill and began cycling down physically. A transplant is the last resort, the only possibility for life after all other avenues have been explored.

I have written this book for three reasons. First, it burst forth, so eager to be told that it almost seemed to write itself. Second, I want to offer what I've learned to others who may be going through their own life-challenging experiences. Third, I wish to honor and express my gratitude to my heart donor, his family, and to donor families everywhere. It is only because of their generous gift that I am alive to write this story.

One

1993

It was November 18, 1993, and dinner was delicious. It was Barry's birthday, and our friend Nino had come to our home in Lafayette, Colorado, to cook with me. Nino's a great cook and the afternoon passed swiftly as we prepared our favorite dishes. I cooked Indian food; he cooked Mexican. What a feast.

Later that night I started wheezing, which was unusual for me. Within moments I could barely breathe. Barry called the doctor and we were told to go immediately to the emergency room. Sara, our daughter, was only five years old at the time and already asleep. Luckily, our neighbor was willing to watch her while we rushed to the nearest hospital. Barry stayed with me in the emergency room until I was transferred by ambulance to University Hospital in Denver. Then he went home to be with Sara. I was scared, lying in that hospital room, not knowing what was happening to me.

I was diagnosed with congestive heart failure (CHF), a condition in which the heart fails to pump blood with normal efficiency, affecting the other organs. My lungs, unable to function normally for lack of blood flow, filled with fluid, a condition known medically as pulmonary edema. The salty dinner seemed to have been the reason for the fluid retention that evening; but the underlying cause, as we were soon to find out, was more serious.

After the drama and fear of the previous evening, just waking up and being alive was ecstasy. When Barry came the next morning we were both struck that, instead of being scared and upset, we felt a measure of grace and peace, which was both inexplicable and undeniable. Of course, grace and peace were not all that we were to feel.

I was hospitalized five days for observation and testing. The most important test was an angiogram, and it was done in the cardiac catheterization lab. It would determine if I had coronary artery disease. A small catheter was inserted into an artery in my groin and guided up to view the arteries of my heart, to see if they were blocked. Dye was inserted so that the arteries could be seen.

Because local anesthesia was used, I was awake during the procedure and I watched the monitor as the dye went into my arteries. My interest in science and my fascination with the technology in that room brought another dimension to the moment. I watched with fascination the inner workings of my body. Dr. Groves, head of the catheterization lab, performed the angiogram. I was relieved to hear him say my blood vessels were as clean as a baby's, but it meant that the cause for my CHF was something else.

Since that first visit to University Hospital I have seen Dr. Groves many times. He's my favorite doctor in that lab. He's confident and highly skilled, and he also shows caring and concern for all his patients.

Test results showed the cause of this episode of congestive heart failure was hypertrophic cardiomyopathy, a thickening of the heart septum (the wall between the right and left sides of the heart) that causes the heart to pump less efficiently, leading to congestive heart failure and, eventually, to death. There is no cure for this disease. Five close family members—my sister, Joanne; my aunt Clara; her two children (Paula and Mel); and Mel's son, Josh—had cardiomyopathy. I was the sixth. Even though medications can alleviate some of the symptoms, such as shortness of breath and fatigue, the heart continues to deteriorate.

Cardiomyopathy carries with it the risk of sudden death from arrhythmias (irregular heart beats). One night while Josh was walking from a parking lot to a restaurant, he collapsed and died. He was twenty-seven years young. He died before I had symptoms—when I thought I never would have symptoms. His loss was devastating; his family's grief deep and long lasting. The possibility that this could happen to me did not escape my awareness.

During my hospitalization, the chief attending cardiologist came to see me. He is fascinated by statistics and research and I respect his extensive knowledge, but he is not known for a sterling bedside manner. I can still see him standing at the foot of my bed.

"You have a condition called cardiomyopathy," he said, "and at this time there is no cure for it. It caused this episode of heart failure. You can expect that within the next ten years, you will need a heart transplant."

I was so shaken that I couldn't speak. For the next two years, I could only refer to the transplant as the "BIG T."

I didn't know anyone with a transplant. The mere thought of such a prospect was shocking and frightening for me, for Barry, and for everyone who knew me. Sara was only five and didn't really understand what we were facing. The possibility of a transplant meant I was dying, but death was an issue for other people, not for me. I wasn't prepared to lose everything—especially not my husband and my daughter. I couldn't imagine Barry as a single father, Sara motherless. I was overwhelmed.

Five days later, when the doctors were convinced I was stable for the time being, I was sent home. I became a regular patient at the heart failure/heart transplant clinic at University Hospital in Denver. I still laugh when I recall my first visit. I walked up to the receptionist and said, "My name is Gaea Shaw and I'm here for the heart success clinic." (I just hated that word "failure"!) The receptionist looked serious, already fried by eight o'clock in the morning. Her head down, she said, "You mean heart fail—." then looked up with a grin. I realize now how blind I kept myself to the obvious fact that the two clinics were together for a purpose and that eventually I would graduate from the heart failure side to the transplant side.

My will to live is strong. Grace and grit, I call it. I was a compliant patient. I went for my doctor's appointments, took many medications, and adhered to a strict low-sodium diet. Cutting out salt to reduce fluid buildup in my body was required in order to maintain some semblance of a normal life, but this wasn't easy because I was addicted to salt.

My main source of support came from my sister and cousins, who had more experience than I did in coping with the disease and medications. They all had strong spirits; it was nurturing to stay in touch with them. My cousin Paula sent me recipes for cooking with low or no salt and teased me about my love of salty chips. I watched myself do something so many of us do. Even though I knew the life-threatening risk I was taking, I still resisted cutting out salt. It took about six weeks and was painfully hard, but I knew my life depended on it. I gave up salt.

I had to bring my own dinner to potlucks because the food brought by the other guests contained salt. I made my own bread with practically no salt, and in general I just kept the salt down to a bland but necessary minimum. Sometimes I was downright angry about the whole thing. But it kept me alive, so I did it.

If I gained weight suddenly from fluid retention I took diuretics, medications to get rid of excess fluid in the body. All the drugs and the dosages needed continual monitoring, and I often felt short of breath, exhausted, weak, or light-headed. Strenuous exercise was out of the question, as it tired me so quickly. In the earlier stages of CHF I could walk a little, but that changed as time went on.

A few years before all this happened I had left teaching and started my own small business as a wedding videographer. I enjoyed shooting weddings and the work was certainly different from teaching. After my hospitalization, however, the only way I could continue running my business was by hiring an assistant to carry all my equipment.

Barry took over more of the housework, grocery shopping, and yard work. He was willing to do whatever had to be done to make my life easier. He never complained, except to express frustration when I overextended myself and ended up exhausted. I remember one doctor telling me during this phase, "Gaea, most people can afford to get exhausted once in a while. You can only afford to get tired." Barry was, simply, devoted and compassionate. He just put one foot in front of the other, so to speak, to make it through those years. Shortly after the transplant, he confessed that for years he checked on me in the middle of the night to see if I was still breathing. It wasn't until after the transplant, when he saw that I was okay, that he gave himself permission to melt into some of his own exhaustion and stress from the years of taking care of me.

We only heard an occasional complaint from Sara that her mommy couldn't do very much. I don't think she really understood the enormity of what was going on until later. Truthfully, I don't think we did either; we just saw my heart slowly deteriorate and took each downward phase as it came. Because Sara is adopted, we were relieved that the legacy of congenital heart disease would not be passed on to her.

In April 1994, less than five months after I was diagnosed with cardiomyopathy, Barry, Sara, and I went to southern California to be with my mother. She had advanced Parkinson's disease and was near the end of her life. My brother, Ron, also has Parkinson's disease. In our family, Parkinson's and cardiomyopathy are the result of a genetic glitch. In other words, those of us with this damaged gene are likely to get one or the other disease.

The visit with my mother was difficult because we knew it was the last time we'd see her. I took some small solace in finding words to express my love and appreciation to her, but saying goodbye was excruciating. If that weren't emotional enough, we got a phone call while we were there that my beloved sister, Joanne (who was in northern California for a dear friend's funeral), had died unexpectedly in the middle of the night. Heartbroken, we drove to Joanne's funeral. My mother, too sick to attend her own daughter's funeral, died two weeks later. I was beside myself with grief. I had just lost the two most influential and dearly loved women in my life.

Joanne had the sudden-death syndrome of cardiomyopathy, a component that my doctors continually searched for in me but never found. It was that aspect of the disease that claimed her life. She had been evaluated for a transplant and decided against it, but she was reconsidering the possibility when she died. I wish she had gotten a transplant before it was too late.

My sister's loss was enormous and grieving took a long time. We have a little antique cabinet in our living room that Barry turned into an altar. It holds Buddha statues, feathers, candles, and other little treasures that have special meaning for each of us. Barry brought out photos of Joanne and my mom and placed them on the altar. It was many months before I was ready to return the photos to their albums.

Time passed, and the only physical change for me was a downward spiral. For the next two years I continued my clinic visits and tried an experimental medication with hopes of reversing or slowing the disease progression, but nothing improved. I became more frail and limited with each passing day. But I was stubborn and wouldn't quit working. One evening in the fall of 1996, while shooting a wedding, I went into atrial fibrillation—irregular, chaotic heartbeats. I was frightened and uncomfortable. My assistant took over and shot the rest of the wedding reception.

The only way to bring my heart back into rhythm was to electrically de-fibrillate (cardiovert) me with those paddles you see in hospital ER programs on TV. But this was no simple deal. The risk of stroke with a defibrillation is high because the procedure could loosen a blood clot and send it to the brain, so I needed to take Coumadin, a blood-thinning medication, for six weeks before the procedure could be done. It was a long six weeks. I could feel my heart beating chaotically in my chest and I felt even more tired and off-balance than usual. I was scared that I might get worse before they could do the procedure. I might even die. And Coumadin is tricky. There had to be weekly monitoring of my blood-clotting ability. If my blood was too thin, I could hemorrhage easily; if it was too thick there was the risk of blood clots. The doctors changed my Coumadin dosage frequently over the six-week period, until my blood was just right.

Finally it was time to have the procedure. Barry and I went to the hospital. I settled into my bed and waited. The doctor came to tell me the risks of the defibrillation: stroke; death; procedure failure which would require more hospitalization and drugs; blood clots, especially in the lungs or legs; allergic reaction to the anesthesia; skin burns from the voltage going through the paddles.

I signed the release form, acknowledging to myself that a stroke was more frightening than death. The procedure was done in my hospital room. The anesthesia contained something that totally blocked memory of the procedure. I think this is done because a patient flatlines (dies, so to speak) for an instant, and such memories could be traumatic. I certainly don't remember anything that happened after the anesthesia took effect. I awoke with paddle burns on my tender chest. The defibrillation was a success and my heart rhythm was back to normal.

1997

Not long after the intensely emotional experience of the defibrillation and all that led up to it, I arrived home from the market so short of breath that I could barely walk the fifteen steps from my car to the house. I sat on the porch and wept. My heart was failing and I was frightened.

In early April of 1997, I had an appointment with the doctor who performed the defibrillation five months earlier. He told me what I already knew: it was time to be evaluated for a transplant. My heart function was very poor and the medications were no longer helping me. I was in end-stage heart failure with, at best, only a forty percent chance of surviving one more year.

I sobbed right there in front of him. Later, he apologized for forgetting I was a person and not just another "heart." My tears reminded him that patients are people first; they are not just body parts. It was a defining moment and certainly the beginning of a more respectful relationship for us both.

Death will come. We all know that. But most of us don't spend much time thinking about it. In fact, most of us design our lives to avoid dealing with death. I was devastated, facing issues that anyone with terminal illness must address. This was not a club I chose to join, but there I was. How could I deal with all that was in front of me? Where would I begin? Was I open to receiving support and, if so, what kind?

I believe all of us have a strong intuitive sense that we tend to ignore. But during that period I felt a huge shift in awareness. I experienced an awakening of intuition and spirit within me, and I found myself on a road moving toward some unknown destiny. I was completely ready for the journey, wherever it led me and however it appeared. I knew it wasn't a journey I could travel alone. But where would I find the emotional, spiritual, and energetic support I needed and what would that mean?

Part of the answer came when I met Melanie Brown, a physical therapist and spiritual healer who sees and works with energy in the body and soul. As the mother of three young children, Melanie understood the issues I was facing about my death. I had many questions: Did I want to go ahead with the transplant or not? What if I decided to have a transplant but died during surgery? What if I survived the surgery but had a miserable quality of life? How would I explain the process to Sara? How could I stay emotionally open to Barry? How would I be able to handle all the medications? How could I get financial and spiritual support? How would I find someone to take care of Sara while I was in the hospital and help for me when I came home?

With Melanie, answers flowed naturally and swiftly. I was encouraged to be authentic, allowing sadness, fear, confidence—whatever appeared—to present itself at any given moment. For someone facing the possibility of death, inviting raw, intimate vulnerability in this way had a huge impact.

I started to see that "healing" didn't necessarily mean my heart would get better or even that I would have a successful transplant. Because the possibility of my death was so great, healing my spirit was the work at hand. If I prayed to heal my body, I might be wasting my time. The surrender started there and continued as we worked together.

Barry and I spent hours discussing options, crying and embracing one another. We decided to have the evaluation. For the next two months, I had lots of tests. If any other organs or body systems were damaged by my failing heart, I would not be eligible for a transplant. The tests were critical and we did not take them lightly. There were ultrasound vascular studies, a VO2 treadmill that measures oxygen levels during exercise, a chest x-ray, a lung function/breathing test, and an electrocardiogram. There was a gated-blood-pool scan (MUGA), in which a radioactive tracer is injected into the veins while a machine takes pictures of the heart to measure how well the ventricles pump blood. There were kidney function studies, blood tests, an abdominal ultrasound, and a right-heart catheterization (a narrow tube is inserted into a large blood vessel in the neck and pushed down to the heart). Information can then be obtained about the heart function, the size of the heart, and any potential problems for the lungs' ability to work with a new heart. A heart biopsy can be performed at the same time. Tiny pieces of the heart are removed and analyzed.

And there was more, including a psychiatric evaluation to determine if I would get the kind of emotional and logistical support needed from family and friends to go through the ordeal of such a major surgery and the enormous challenges following it. Would I be compliant and vigilant about taking the fifteen or so life-sustaining medications needed every day post-transplant? Was I emotionally stable enough to handle all the uncertainties of such a major life change?

Barry was evaluated, too, to determine his ability to provide the support I would need. The finance division at the hospital ascertained whether our insurance would pay for the transplant, treatment, and medications. Finally, a social worker met with me for about three hours and asked a million questions, none of which I can remember.

The tests were extremely stressful and it was a scary time, but I was placed on the heart transplant waiting list in late May 1997.

While all of this was happening with me, my cousin Mel went into cardiac arrest at his doctor's office, was "paddled" back to life, and rushed to the hospital. With death imminent and no other options available, he decided to have a heart transplant. After a six-week wait in the hospital for a donor heart, he received a great one. He has faced many medical challenges since his transplant, but his heart has remained true and steady since the first day.

Mel was a tremendous inspiration and valuable resource, once I passed all the tests. He alerted and prepped me about what to expect from the side effects of transplant medications, especially the steroids I would be taking, and told me how much more alive I'd feel after the transplant. Mel's gift of humor in the face of adversity shone through even then. What a blessing!

The stark reality of facing a transplant brought my video business to an abrupt halt. I wasn't working much by then anyway. I couldn't. I had been stubborn, as sick as I was, trying to climb church steps and walk around the countryside to videotape weddings.

We decided to wait until mid-June to be put on a transplant waiting list. I could have been listed right away, but Sara was going to Girl Scout camp in June and we didn't want to get a call that there was a heart for me while she was away. So we waited.

The waiting list is composed of two parts. Those waiting in the hospital are called status one. I was well enough to wait at home, so I was status two. I needed a heart that matched my blood type and size; if a donor's heart weren't a match for a status-one person, it would go the status-two list and possibly to me, depending on my placement on that list. We were told it would probably be four to eight months before we would get the call that they had a donor heart for me. Barry and I each had pagers, and we were available twenty-four hours a day for that call.

How does one find the strength to face all of this—the possibility of death, a high-risk surgery, a complicated and unknown lifestyle after the transplant if I did survive it, concerns about my family and the potential loss they might endure? I'm talking about facing the unknown. So many of us live under the illusion that we know what our future will be. The truth is, any one of us could be dead in the next second from a freak accident, a stroke, a fatal car crash—regardless of how healthy we are. Who can know for certain when death will come?

I had a lifetime habit of worry and fear. My parents lived through the Depression, so worrying about money was part of the air I lived and breathed. As an adult I carried that same worry, fearing that I wouldn't have enough money to survive until the next month. This was in spite of the fact that I had earned a teacher's salary and then ran my own business. I had not made a lot of money, but I was certainly far from homeless. One day I admitted to Barry that every single day of my life I felt anxious. Usually it was about money, but any issue could be added to my worry list. That same day I also acknowledged the truth: I had always managed financially. The worry was eating me up and it was a lie. From that day on, I have essentially been free of money concerns. I don't have more money now than when I was worrying about it all the time, but the worry that gnawed at me continually is gone. Oh yes, I still have my moments, but they don't last. They don't stick.

Now I had something real to worry about: my life, a transplant, and death. Moving from fear and worry as a way of life to the trust and surrender that is now constantly at my side, evolved over time with Melanie's help. I also had the guidance of a wonderful woman, Gangaji, an American who met her teacher in India. Barry remembers the exact date we met her—October 2, 1992—because of her impact on our lives. The value of all spiritual teachers—of whatever faith—is their ability to lead each of us to our true nature. Gangaji did that by pointing me to an inner observer that watches all I see and feel, turbulent or not. This observer has no problem with anything that comes and goes. The "icky" stuff still shows up from time to time, but it does not stick because I am more connected to who I really am rather than to my mental spin. By letting go of all my ideas of who I think I am,

I have experienced a death of sorts. By being still, going endlessly deeper and deeper, what I have found is indescribably beautiful and never-ending. It is my essence. It is peace.

Being human, I have moments of abandoning this essence. When I do, my suffering is immediate. When the transplant issue showed up, I had the opportunity to look at death, my fears, my attachments, and I found, amazingly yet not surprisingly, peace. When a bout of fear shows up again, I just check inside and notice that the peace has not gone anywhere.

The transplant and the journey it took me on are the greatest gifts I ever received because I found trust, peace, surrender, community, and lots of love. Some people can experience all of that without the benefit of a teacher or guide or a life-threatening experience. For me, I am grateful that guidance showed up in my life and that I was ready to receive it.

This was an awesome process and I was amazed to be going through it. Barry and I were being led by grace and mysterious reservoirs of strength, courage, and undying faith. After all our questions were answered and lists were made, there was still the enormous unknown, what I called "the God realm." Barry pointed out that everything is the God realm.

Sara spent a lot of time with her friends, which gave Barry and me the time and luxury to be with each other. Looking into one another's eyes we needed no words. Love flowed between us.

All my life, I have been self-sufficient, rarely asking for help. With so much at stake, it was time to change all that. I challenged myself to write a letter to my friends and family requesting their support. I also created a phone tree so that when the big event came everyone would be notified with a minimum of effort on our part. Little did I know what would happen when I sent that letter.

June 8, 1997
Dear Friends and Family,

   Some of you have not heard from me for a while, and others are in constant contact, so this is a general letter to all, and

I hope it bridges the gap for those of you who are ever in my heart, even if we don't talk or write frequently.

I have been having heart problems. The condition is cardiomyopathy, and its active form is heart failure. Since I was first hospitalized, I have been on a slew of medications that have helped me live a semblance of a normal life, even though my baseline of activity has lowered steadily. My heart has been deteriorating, and lately, severely. So. My big news is that I am going to have a heart transplant.

I will be listed officially on June 26, 1997, and can be called any time to come to the hospital when a match is found. This call could come in days, weeks, or months. Barry and I will both have pagers for only this call. When the call comes, we'll need to get Sara and leave for the hospital immediately. If the thoroughly checked-out donor heart is indeed a good match, then the surgery will happen. If it isn't a good match, we'll have to deal with the adrenaline rush and disappointment until the next pager beep. This doesn't happen all the time, but we have been warned about it.

When I was told that an evaluation for a transplant was the next step (there is no other medical option at this point) I wept a lot, both in the doctor's office and at home. Barry was and continues to be a major support and dear friend, holding me and talking with me all hours of the days and nights.

I have found a champion in Melanie Brown, a spiritual energy healer who works with people facing life-threatening illness. Although death is inevitable, in our culture that reality is something most of us avoid. I discovered that by looking directly at that possibility came the deepest—and continually deepening—peace of my life. I keep checking in with myself to see if I am in some kind of denial, and I am quite sure that I am not. Don't misunderstand me, there are many rocky moments when fears and dread arise, but they come as part of a flowing river and pass, until the next time they reappear. I am seeing the value of living in truth each moment. This allows me not to take a stand but to be fluid with what comes and goes.

Barry is experiencing the same peace—the kind where everything shows up. To go through this process consciously, individually, and as a family is true healing. Sara finally asked some questions and initiated a discussion. We did our best to answer her questions truthfully in a vocabulary that a nine year old could understand. I feel relieved that she knows the truth and understands it. What a blessing for us, to be with God in all of this.

A heart transplant no longer has the high risk that it once did. I'm confidant that I'll survive the surgery and difficult recovery, and will have energy and vitality again that has been missing for a long time. I look forward to having the energy to hike, ride a bike, be an active mom, and work. Barry has been carrying the financial responsibility here for a while, and as we were a two-income family, things have been quite tight.

We have two weeks to get ourselves organized, to get support systems in place, and to figure out the logistics for the time of surgery and after. Recovery normally takes about three months if all goes well, and it will be six months or longer before I can return to some kind of work.

We will need support when I return home from the hospital. Coverage for Sara, some home-cooked meals, driving me down to the hospital for my clinic visits, money for my expensive medications—these are some of the requests we're making to you. We would also love your support in the form of prayers and/or your special brand of heartfelt wishes. If you can, imagine us surrounded by healing light.

Whether you help in some tangible way or not, we know that your thoughts and prayers are with us. We feel blessed to have such loving friends in our life. Thank you for everything.

Much love,
Gaea, Barry, and Sara

Within days the calls and letters started coming. Someone took charge of coverage for Sara. Meals were organized for us upon my return from the hospital. One friend arranged transportation for my many visits to Denver for doctor appointments and rehabilitation. A friend planned a successful fundraiser; about three hundred people came. There was live music, a catered reception donated by some of my wedding business colleagues, and a raffle of donated items from twenty local businesses. Strangers as well as old friends were there to support me as the focal point, but really it was a celebration of our one heart. Over $6,000 in donations was collected that night. Barry and I came home, sat on the bed with the box of money, and gleefully counted all those ones, tens, and twenties.

At our bank, another "angel" spearheaded an effort to raise money and it poured in. The greatest surprise and my biggest lesson was that people were thrilled to help and thanked us for the opportunity to serve. I had no idea of the power and enormity of support that would come from opening my heart and asking for help.

I enjoyed a sweet summer with Sara, rich in love and deep connection. We spent time together not "doing," just hanging out at the house or running a few errands. To prepare her for the transplant day, we all went down to the hospital one afternoon. I wanted Sara to see where I'd have surgery and what the intensive care unit (ICU) was like. When we left she asked me if people die when they get a transplant. I told her yes, but more people lived, and I planned to be one of them.

We had some good talks in the car. When it felt right, I gave her some "feeling" vocabulary and asked if it fit. One day I said, "What a wonderful summer I'm having with you, Sara! I wonder if it's partly because we both know this big surgery is coming soon and it makes our time together seem more precious." I started crying. She agreed and then, as was natural for that nine year old, she went right on to the next subject!

Days passed. I became aware of fear and resistence brewing inside me. Sometimes I felt like I was watching a play where the lead character would remove her stage makeup after the third act and go home. Was I really so sick that I would elect to have a heart transplant? It felt bizarre. What if recovery weren't smooth? Would I face months of hell?

One day I took my fears to Melanie. She helped me trace them back to seeing my friend Tom the previous week. He was four months post heart transplant and very sick from all the steroids and anti-rejection medications. Interestingly, he was still filled with gratitude and the blessings of his new heart. In my fear, I focused on those same drugs I would have to take after the transplant. Melanie said something I've never forgotten. "God provides all, including the drugs you'll need to take. If you don't shift your perspective to welcome the life-saving aspect of the drugs, you'll undermine yourself." As she spoke, I felt the shift once again back to ease, peace, acceptance, and gratitude.

I decided to hide some gifts for Barry and Sara in my hospital bag and present them at the hospital just before my surgery. I bought Barry a beaded necklace that included a beaded leather pouch containing a crystal. I wanted to get Sara her first charm bracelet. This would be a fitting mother-daughter gift, one to remember me by if I didn't survive and one that we could continue adding to, if I lived.

At my neighborhood jewelry store I explained my medical situation, about needing the transplant, having a nine-year-old daughter, and how special this gift would be.

I looked at the bracelets and a lovely angel charm and told the jeweler that I didn't think I could afford them just yet, but I would return soon if I changed my mind. Another customer, a young woman I didn't know, overheard my story and asked if I'd let her pay for the first charm. She said that so many people had helped her and her daughter that it just felt right to do the same for Sara, even though she didn't know us.

I was deeply moved and tears welled up in my eyes. The thought came, "Oh, no, I couldn't accept that. I don't even know you." Then I just "stepped out of my own way" and let her buy the charm.

Most of us are better at giving than receiving. In the jewelry store I learned that receiving graciously is actually a gift for the giver. I don't know the woman's name and she didn't want further contact. She just wanted to give me a gift. What an opportunity. What a moment.

In September 1997, autumn wasn't providing the only change. Mother Theresa and Princess Diana died, reminding me and the rest of the world that dear ones live forever only in our hearts.

I sensed a quickening of the transplant process. I awakened one day knowing that I would be saying goodbye to my physical heart, that I would be getting a call from the hospital soon. They would remove my ailing old heart and give me another. It was a quiet, inward, powerful time.

Some of our friends couldn't believe I wasn't afraid. They thought I was in denial. But I was so much in the moment that I truly did feel peace and God's grace. I imagined that fear would probably arise when I got "the call," when I was at the hospital, or certainly after the surgery. But at that moment, I was grateful for the peace.

Barry saw his own fears and concerns, how he was being tough, feeling that somehow it was his responsibility whether I lived or not. What an impossible belief. After we discussed it, he asked for and got support—massages, time off, visits with friends. It was great to see him taking care of himself.

We spent quiet time together after Sara was asleep. I watched my tendency to go inward and not talk when I was upset, and I promised to communicate better. It brought more aliveness to our relationship. It was wonderful.

By the end of September I was feeling vulnerable, young, and scared. I realized that doctors would be taking over my entire physical body and well-being. I predicted that my new heart would come soon, and I wrote a letter to my steadily failing heart.

Dear Heart,

I bow in gratitude for how you have served me for so very long. I owe my life to you. You have been with me from my first moment. Through everything, for all these years. I feel deeply that you are ready for retirement, and that you support my search for another heart. Thank you for staying with me until it's time for a new heart to join me. Tell the new heart not to fear. It will have been a loyal servant to some other being before me. I will welcome it and do whatever I can to ease its transition to its new home, here. I honor you, my beloved heart. I will never forget you. You will live in my true heart forever. God Bless.

Two

October 1997

There was quite a blizzard on Saturday, October 25, 1997. Two hundred cars were stranded on the road to the Denver International Airport, hundreds of flights were cancelled. Doctors were flown in by helicopter to the hospital. Roads were closed everywhere. We settled in for the duration. Sara's friend Hanna was visiting and stayed with us two nights because there was no way to take her home. Barry gave up his attempts to clear the driveway and make a path for the car because all the roads were blocked. We discussed how ironic it would be if we got the call and weren't able to drive the thirty-five miles to the hospital. Would we call the police? the fire department? Barry said not to worry, because even the doctors were having such a hard time getting to the hospital that probably nothing would happen. I felt very peaceful. In fact, our entire home was filled with grace and peace that night. It was very palpable, very sweet.

The next day we awakened to bright sunshine. Typical of Colorado, severe blizzards can be followed the next day by bright sun and temperatures warm enough to start the meltdown. Barry went out immediately to clear a path for the car. We all went to the supermarket, where we laughed, thinking the whole population of the town was there, enjoying their first chance to get out in two days.

Halfway out of the parking lot my pager beeped. Because we previously had had some false alarms with wrong numbers, I withheld any response until I saw the number on the pager. I knew that number. It was the hospital. "This is it," I said. "This is the call."

The closest pay phone was only a few yards away at the Burger King on the corner. "I have an emergency," I said to the man using it. He ignored me, so I rushed inside and told the workers I needed their phone. I'm sure the look on my face conveyed the seriousness of the moment. They let me come behind the counter and I called the hospital. The line was busy! After three tries, I gave up.

"Let's just go home," I told Barry. "We're only seven minutes away and we can try again."

We headed home. One mile from the house, in front of our neighborhood gas station, we were paged again. The attendant was outside shoveling snow. We pulled in and, without asking, I went behind the counter and used the phone. This time we got through.

Nancy, one of the transplant coordinators, answered. "We have a heart," she said, "and at this point it's looking very good. There are more tests needed, but we'd like you to come down to the hospital. Take your time. We'll see you in a few hours."

So home we went. It took us only twenty minutes to get ready. My bag was already packed. We called Hanna's house but nobody was home. Another friend came to get her. We activated the phone tree with over eighty names by making the first three calls (see appendix 5, page 93). Everyone soon heard that the process had begun.

How can I begin to describe our emotions at this time? We were excited to the max—and nervous and scared. Yet at the same time, I was very focused and quite calm. This dive into the unknown came exactly four months after I was placed on the transplant waiting list.

We drove on half-cleared roads and highways to the hospital. We were there by noon. I checked in, and we waited.

The surgery was not assured, as there was much to determine about the condition of the donor's heart. Nevertheless, I was medically prepped as if the transplant were going to happen. The nurse inserted an IV line, I was given high doses of anti-rejection steroids, took an antibacterial shower, wasn't allowed any food or drink, and we waited. Blood was drawn both for routine tests and a final cross match with the donor. I took a chest x-ray and EKG, was given a medical history and physical exam, and met with an anesthesiologist. While all of this was happening, I was excited, joyous, and feeling ready for a new heart.

The phone tree we created worked. While the nurses prepared me for possible surgery, seven dear friends came and stayed to support all of us, especially Barry and Sara, through the event. All of these friends are deeply steeped in spirit, and they held a holy vigil through it all. Melanie, my spiritual healer, and Karin, a dear friend and also a powerful healer, were part of the group. Sara was also there, of course. Our discussions, the visits to the ICU, and previous introductions to doctors helped prepare her for this day.

From my bed I had a beautiful view of the Denver skyline and the Rocky Mountains to the west. I kept telling everyone how beautiful the sunset was, with the sky bathed in varied shades of orange and red. Because they were facing me instead of the window, they were missing it. Melanie thought I was wondering if it would be my last sunset. Actually, I was feeling enormous trust, surrender, and confidence.

At about 9:00 that night we were all sitting with eyes closed, silent and meditative. I heard someone enter the room, opened my eyes, and saw a doctor looking at us. He introduced himself as the surgeon, Dr. David Campbell, and said, "Yes, it's a go." He was going with a team of doctors to procure the heart and bring it back. Surgery would be at about 11:00 p.m.

I am teary even now as I write this, seeing how my life changed at that very moment: knowing I was so close to death and being given a second chance at life. There was profound grace for me and everyone else in that room.

Soon after Dr. Campbell brought us the good news, I was taken down to the final pre-op room, with my entourage in tow. I met Kathi, the OR—operating room—nurse who would communicate with Barry during the operation. I asked her to make positive statements to me during the operation. I didn't want to put words in her mouth; I just wanted her verbal support. Because I imagined that in the coma-like state I'd be in after surgery I might not know if I were alive or dead, I asked Barry to tell me repeatedly, once I arrived in the intensive care unit, that everything had gone well.

Finally, it was time. The gurney arrived, nurses, technicians, and all. Everyone hugged me. Barry, Sara, and I hugged last, with explosions of tears that occur again as I write this. They walked beside me to the last allowable door, and then I was on my way. It was a very emotional moment, facing the unknown and the possibility that we might never see each other again. I was crying as they wheeled me away, hearing Sara sobbing in the background. I am especially grateful to my friend Karen Mohr, who arrived just after I was taken into surgery. I learned later that she and Sara connected deeply that night. Karen took Sara under her wing and gave her the nurturing she needed. I also heard from the others who were there that, concerned as Barry was about me, he took plenty of time to hold and comfort Sara.

The universe sent me the right OR nurse. When I arrived in the operating room, Kathi held my hand and said, "Gaea, this room and everything in it, is filled with Divine Grace. Feel the Grace within you." With words like that I knew that I was in the very best of hands. The surgery went more quickly than usual and I lost no blood at all, unusual for heart transplant surgery.

Kathi called Barry in the waiting room throughout the surgery—when the incision was made, when my old heart was removed, when the new heart was in, when I was being sewn up, and when surgery was complete. Barry was grateful for her kindness and clear communication. The operation took only three-and-one-half hours. There were no complications and it went incredibly well.

After surgery I was taken to the ICU and put on a respirator—a tube attached to a breathing machine was put down my throat—and my hands were restrained so that I wouldn't pull out the tube. I can still hear Barry's voice saying softly, "Gaea, you did great. You have a new heart, the vibrant heart of a fifteen-year-old boy." He said it many times and I heard him, but of course I couldn't respond. When I started to awake I heard the nurses shouting that when I could keep my eyes open, they would take out the breathing tube. How I worked to get those eyes open! Finally I succeeded. Sometime that evening the breathing tube was removed.

I was in intensive care for five days but I don't remember most of what happened. There were visits from friends and the nurses on the heart failure team who had cared for me for so many years. I have no memory of any of that. I remember only two things from those five days: Barry's loving voice and frequent, violent, uncontrollable shaking. The most likely explanation for the shaking was that I was in shock from the surgery. By the time I was ready to move to the transplant ward, the shaking had ended and I was relatively coherent.

My first awareness, as I was regaining some sense of myself, was that I had strong life energy surging through me. There I was, so beat up from transplant surgery, tubes coming out of me everywhere, barely able to move, yet I was aware of this incredible change. Life force!

Reports from Transplant Night

While I was having my chest cracked open, my old heart removed and a new heart put in, Barry, Sara, and our friends who were at the hospital that night had their own intense experiences.

Barry's Report:

> *Gaea had just been taken to the OR around midnight. Sara, our friends, and I went up to the fourth-floor ICU waiting room to settle in for the night and early morning. We joined other families who were also waiting and not knowing. Everybody in that room was uncertain of the outcome of their loved one's ordeal. The energy in the room was highly charged with the*

edges of life and death teeter-tottering every minute with every new report from doctors, nurses, and OR updates.

For our group of nine, much was happening. Sara was still distraught from saying goodbye to Momma ten minutes ago. She was tearful and broken-hearted, full of love and uncertainty. My friend Karen Mohr, who has such a deep angelic and compassionate nature, cradled Sara with natural warmth that was both comforting and honoring to Sara. Karen held her and let her grieve, thank God. She put blankets on Sara's cold, shaky body, and she stayed by her side the entire duration of Gaea's surgery. Sara settled in and I was never out of her sight nor out of arms' reach. Karen offered the mothering that Sara needed. I took everything in and yet was very still and focused on Gaea.

One of the attending nurses in the OR with Gaea that night was Kathi. She told us that she would be calling me at every major step of Gaea's heart transplant, updating me with Gaea's status. The crucial points of reference were: the opening incision into the chest wall and breaking of the sternum, taking the heart out and putting Gaea on a heart bypass machine, putting the prepared new heart in and defibrillating it (electrically shocking it into beating, starting), seeing that the heart was successfully beating, sewing Gaea up and finalizing the surgical transplant, and, finally, wheeling Gaea to ICU where I could, in time, be with her.

I sat by the phone in the ICU waiting room where Kathi would call me. This was my hitching post, my seat of prayer throughout Gaea's surgery. The rest of the group stayed close and found their own spot alone or with others in deep prayer, meditation, holding hands, or coming to be with me. There was a sacred bond of unity and undying support amongst us all. This sacred love, pure intention of wellness and light, directed at Gaea, was enormous. It filled the whole room.

After every call from Kathi I would report back to the group as we huddled together. A few moments were spent together, and then everybody would return to their way of being with Gaea and each other. *The* dynamic was beautiful—we were alone yet very together.

Prior to her surgery, a healer, Melanie Brown, who is also a physical therapist, had helped Gaea. Her strong, quiet presence exudes faith and confidence. Throughout the night she worked energetically both with Gaea, her donor, and the donor's family. She has the God-given facility to channel healing energy flow as well as to intuitively pick up information that can be both insightful and of the highest service. Melanie was a vital presence with our group that night.

Another good friend of ours, Karin Aarons, was there, as was her husband and our dear friend, Ron. Karin, too, is a healer, teacher, and medicine woman. She and Melanie know each other and teamed up that night, doing their own unique form of receiving and exchanging messages, coming together for Gaea's highest good and affecting us all with their profound gifts.

Two other dear friends were there to support me— Chaitanya and Sheldon. The two of them and Ron connected and shared throughout the surgery, and their presence rounded out the richness of the group that night.

What a night. Under the circumstances, it couldn't have been more perfect. Nothing will ever be the same, make no mistake about it. This indelibly changes one's perspective far beyond what we think we know.

Most information about organ donors is withheld out of respect for the donor's family, but we were told that Gaea's donor was a fifteen-year-old boy who had lived in the mountains. We were allowed to know that much.

This dimly lit, huge waiting room, my wife being cut open, saying goodbye to the only heart she had known and which had served her well. . . . Her heart put in a jar—gone—a fifteen-year-old boy dead—suddenly—and Gaea breathing with his unforeseen gift. Would she survive the surgery? Would the heart sustain itself, beating on its own when zapped with those defibrillating paddles? How—when—what—waiting—praying—all a great mystery, a holy ordeal—the deepest surrender of my life. The love of the group, the OR nurse Kathi, Dr. Campbell, Sara by my side, faith and God, and a whole host of angels and guides, holding my hand, all the way through.

We got the last call—the big one—just three-and-one-half hours after the surgery first began. All was well, very good for now. Two unusual occurrences happened during the surgical procedure: Gaea lost no blood and the surgery flew by much faster than expected. There were no roadblocks; great flow and ease were reported.

Kathi told me that the next call I'd be receiving would be from ICU telling me that I could come in and be with Gaea. We all silently celebrated the news. Some of my friends were so tired that they lay on the floor, curled up in blankets, and slept for an hour or two.

At 6:30 or 7:00 a.m. everybody started to make their way home, all making sure that I could handle the aloneness. I assured them all that I was ready and expressed my utter appreciation of their immense support. I needed and welcomed this alone time with Sara. Soon she would be picked up by her friend's mom and taken back to their home. Gaea had prearranged all of this. Sara would be spending four or five nights and days with various friends and their parents, and she would be driven down to the hospital for visits while I stayed with Gaea full time. After lots of hugs and reassurance that Mom was doing well, she left. Sara was so present throughout all of this. What an ordeal and test of faith for a nine year old.

There I was—no sleep—very tearful, wired, scared, surrendered, full of every emotion possible; stripped to the bare-naked vulnerability that wrestled with nothing. I simply sat in vast awe of everything that had transpired. Now the crucial forty-eight hours after surgery had begun. Every minute

I sat holding the hand of Grace, merging with God's will and wisdom into this next excursion into the unknown.

I went in to see Gaea. There must have been seventeen tubes coming out of her. She was on a respirator for breathing. There were chest tubes, catheters, IV's galore, telemetry machines tracking vitals and heart rate, and a pacemaker pacing her new heart that wasn't strong enough yet to beat on its own. I did not recoil—I embraced the totality of what I saw. Gaea was out for the first twelve hours post-surgically. She had asked me beforehand to tell her that she was doing well and to play Bach and Mozart music for her. So I did just that. I placed a set of headphones on her, turned the tape deck on low volume, and excitedly and repeatedly said to her, "Gaea, you're doing great! You have a beautiful new heart—a fifteen-year-old boy's beautiful heart—Gaea, Gaea!" She never blinked an eye—she was totally out. I kissed her forehead, held and stroked her hands, stayed as long as I wasn't in the nurses' way, and visited two to three times an hour, twenty-four hours a day, for five straight days. This was so comforting to me.

In between those visits with Gaea, my time was spent on the phone with friends and relatives, and being with friends who came to see me and bring me food.

I slept a maximum of two hours a day, totaling ten to twelve hours of sleep in five days. On the sixth day, Gaea's heart started to pace on its own. I knew then that it was time for me to go home, reconnect with Sara on Halloween night, and touch base with the reality of life outside the hospital. On the way, I stopped at a market in my neighborhood and bumped into someone I knew. I broke down big time—tears galore—feeling a whole new wave of the enormity of Gaea's, Sara's, and my journey. Gaea was still lying in a hospital bed, and I was breathing real live fresh air with people going about the business of life. I was excited about seeing Sara before she went trick-or-treating. We spent some time together, and again she spent the night with friends, as my plan was to return to the hospital by 6 or 7 a.m. the next day.

I arrived the next morning to see Gaea alive, alert, and beaming. She was moving from ICU to the transplant ward. She had graduated! It was a big leap and kind of a shock that it happened so soon.

That's when everything changed from the life-and-death feel of ICU to the first stages of "you made it." Cardiac rehabilitation and more relaxed nursing slowly began. Only a few IV's remained, along with a zipper-like incision from the first rib area down through the centerline of Gaea's sternum. Here was Gaea, feeling life force surge through her as never before. What a bittersweet edge also, thinking about the death of her donor and his family's devastation. Both the exhaustion and exuberance were evident. The celebration had truly begun.

My brother flew in from California to be with all of us. His loving presence gave me support and brotherly companionship. It was great.

The rest, of course, is Gaea's story. "Thanks" barely scratches the depth of that week's experience.

Sara was almost fourteen when she wrote this, but she was nine that night at the hospital.

Sara's Report:

It was a bitter-cold day; everything was white. The snow crunched under the tires of our car as we drove down the snow-packed street toward the market. It was the day after the big blizzard in October 1997, the 26th to be exact, a weekend. Hanna, my best friend since second grade, was sitting next to me in my dad's old Honda. We were just nine years old, with matching haircuts that hung down to our chins. We laughed as my dad told us jokes only fourth-graders could find funny.

My mom, occupying the front seat of the car, just looked at Dad and smiled. I could tell she was exhausted. She put forth a great deal of energy to be with us this morning; she always wanted to be the best mom that she could, even though she was so sick. She wanted to join in the conversation, but she was too tired to even make a joke. She was suffering from end-stage heart disease and was waiting for a heart transplant. I knew she was worried about this, and we didn't know when we were going to find an organ donor and get the call to go to the hospital. She didn't show her worry; she just smiled because she was always a happy person no matter what.

There was such a happy mood in the car. There were hardly any cars on the road; all you saw was white cold snow all around! But it was warm inside the car and Hanna and I were talking about who we were going to invite to our next birthday parties. I heard a beeping, and my mom turned and looked at my dad. She gave him a very intense stare. I could tell his heart had skipped a beat when he heard the pager go off.

"This is it, Barry," my mom said with an excited yet nervous tone in her voice. Hanna looked confused, curious, and frightened all at once, but I knew exactly what had happened. So many thoughts were rushing through my mind at that moment, and I knew that my family's and my life were about to change forever.

My dad said sternly, "We need to find a phone!" He swerved the station wagon into the King Sooper's parking lot, searching desperately for a pay phone. My parents jumped out of the car, even my tired mother, and raced for the pay phones near Burger King. I was alone in the car with Hanna. I told her that my mom had been paged by the hospital, which meant that they had her new heart waiting at the hospital.

Hanna knew that my mom had been waiting for a heart transplant for about four months now and that it would be an enormous deal when the time came, which was now! We were all so excited, yet we all knew deep down that this wasn't a simple procedure and that there was a chance that my mom wouldn't make it. It was at that point that I realized how much

I loved my mom and how much she had been there for me and loved me.

Outside, I couldn't hear what my dad was saying. I could only see the cloud-like puffs of hot air against the chilly morning coming out of his mouth when he opened it. I could tell he was frustrated. They had to contact the hospital as soon as possible. There was only one pay phone, which was being used by a tall lean man who looked to be in his late twenties. He was leaning against the phone with a cigarette in his hand. He looked as if he were going to take his time, not knowing that my mom had such an emergency. My father was furious; my mother was standing next to him. I could tell by her motions that she was telling him to calm down.

Hanna and I really didn't know what to say to each other at that moment, so we didn't say anything. I just sat there, absorbing everything that was happening. I didn't cry, but I felt sadness inside because I knew the risks that were about to take place very shortly in someone's life whom I loved so dearly. A small tear trickled down my face, but I caught it and wiped it before anyone saw it. My parents hurried back into the still car with big grins across their faces.

"Your mother's getting a new heart tonight, Sara!" my dad exclaimed. I thought, now that's not a phrase every nine-year-old girl gets to hear! We all celebrated in the car, hollering and praising.

My mom was getting a second chance at life! This was one of the happiest days of my life. I loved my mom so much and, no matter what happened later that night, she would always be my mom.

We got in and went to the waiting room. It was morning. We talked to the doctor. He said they had the heart and they had to check it out first. We waited until night and she still hadn't gone into surgery. I did puzzles while we waited.

Finally, they gave my mom medicine and prepared her. She was funny. She forgot to take off her undies, and went to the bathroom to take them off. When she came out of the bathroom, she twirled the undies on her finger and did the hula. Everyone was laughing. Then she started to get tired. She lay down on a bed with all these needles and tubes in her arms. Soon they came and said, "It's time." We all said our goodbyes, not knowing if we'd ever see her again.

My dad and I were very scared. We really cried. I could barely swallow because I was crying so much. Everyone hugged my dad and me. It was around midnight. We went upstairs to get some rest. It wasn't very comfortable because there were only wooden chairs. But I didn't care because I couldn't stop thinking about how my mom was doing. Karen Mohr came by and sat with me for a while. She smelled good, and she reminded me of my mom.

The nurse came up and said mom was doing better than they expected and that she'd be out in about four hours. Three hours passed and they said they finished the surgery. It had gone an hour quicker than it was supposed to, and there was no bleeding. I went to sleep and woke up to the smell of muffins. It was a sunny morning. Everyone was eating breakfast. I asked my dad how Mom was, and he said she was great.

I couldn't wait to see her, but my dad said that I couldn't for a while because she was in the ICU. I went to my friend's house and spent the night. A few days later I asked again if I could see my mom. Dad said no, because she would look too scary. I spent Halloween night trick-or-treating with my friends, and I stayed with different friends for a few nights, because Dad stayed at the hospital.

Finally I got to see her. She didn't look so scary anymore. They had removed the breathing tube and she could only whisper. We visited her for a long time. She was very tired and I could just remember her doing the hula before she went into surgery.

She looked more alive now, more colorful, and chubbier than before. I went home to sleep in my house for the first night in a long time. Dad was really happy and so was I. But my mom didn't come home yet.

We planned to surprise her with a big king-size bed when she came back, but they delivered the bed after she came home because she came home early. That summer, we had a big party celebrating her new heart. All my friends and the people who stayed with us that night at the hospital came.

Now she's much better. She can take long walks and go faster than my dad, our dog Tara, and me.

Although I was still a child, I knew that for my mom to have gotten her heart meant that someone, somewhere, had died and their organs had been donated. I felt such grief for this person's family and friends. I wondered how he or she had died, if they had any pain—and I wondered if their family knew, if they had any family at all, what a positive thing was happening out of their tragedy.

Ron Aarons is a friend who came to support the three of us during the night of the transplant.

Ron's Report:

"We're waiting for the final word, then we will go to see if the heart is right for you." They will be leaving soon. Two doctors will go get the heart. They're not the only ones going. Other teams are preparing to transplant others of the donor's organs. Maybe lungs, liver? People waiting, slowly dying, praying for organs. Another dying and in that death, a hero for others. A meeting of incomprehensible destiny.

The doctors leave; we wait. Barry is nervous, scared, restless, trying to find some way to control the uncontrollable. The doctors call. It's a suitable heart! The operation is on. This is it. It's a go. What do I feel? Happy, scared, excited? Stunned.

I hold Gaea's hand. She's strong, ready. Clear. She has faith. We all go down to the pre-operation staging area, a huge area with empty beds and no personnel. It's nighttime already. It's hard to wait.

Sara is beautiful, loving, real, staying close to her mom. She's been told that her mother may not survive. What is she thinking? What are any of us thinking? This could be our last moment with Gaea.

They're ready. They're coming for Gaea. Now wheeling her bed away. This is it. We walk beside her, each saying little things. I think I say, "Remember Ramana Maharshi," an Indian spiritual master whose works we both studied. Doctors and nurses in green scrubs. We can't go any further. They take Gaea through the terrible swinging doors beyond our reach.

They're going to take her into the operating room, they will open her chest, take out her heart. A machine will pump her blood, oxygenating it, keeping her alive. Then they will bring in the donor's heart, a young vibrant heart, put it in her chest, meticulously sewing it in. They will try to get it to beat. It might not start. They'll keep trying.

Chaitanya has been a friend for years and came to support all of us, but especially Barry.

Chaitanya's Report:

It is about surrender, surrender to what is. Few of us have the opportunity to be in the presence of one in total surrender to life as it presents itself to us. When "disaster" appears, whether it be personal or tribal, a death in the family or a devastating hurricane that wipes out many lives, the usual reaction is to move away from the truth, out of the eye and directly into the raging storm of mind and emotions. It is rare to find someone who has the willingness to stop in the face of this, to surrender to the unbelievable, to the unknown, to live in the clear certainty of this day perhaps being one's last. This is the opportunity of Gaea.

In late June of '97, she and her husband received beepers that would call them to be at University Hospital in Denver within the hour. One day in July, as I was leaving their home, I told Barry that I wanted to be at the hospital to support him during the operation.

As the months of waiting passed, I watched Gaea's stillness, her embrace of what was to come, deepen. She became a home for stillness, for peace. No matter what arose—the fear, the grief, the rage, the incomprehension—there was this stillness in her, which never left.

Near the end of October, I was housesitting for two friends in Longmont, Colorado, the neighboring town to where Barry, Gaea, and Sara lived.

The day before, the metropolitan Denver area was hit by a sudden storm, one for which it was hugely unprepared. Dozens of cars were stranded on the road to the airport, some people trapped there for the better part of the day as nearly three feet of snow was dumped on some areas in less than forty-eight hours. I spent all day Saturday nesting in the house while the storm raged.

Sunday emerged bright and sunny. I headed out to a local coffee shop for a morning brew. Long's Peak glistened with a new coat in the distance, above an expanse of white fields. I left the shop and headed home for another day of hibernation. Approaching the front door, I had the distinct sense that there would be a message on the machine from Barry, alerting me to a call from the hospital. I went directly to the machine, pushed playback, and heard his voice. It was true. Today was the day. The moment had arrived. Everything stopped, all plans, all thoughts. I fed the cats and was quickly in my car, headed for the highway to Denver.

When I arrived at Gaea's hospital room, only her husband and daughter were there with her, but we were soon joined by Melanie Brown, the psychic healer who had been working with her in preparation for the transplant, and Karin Aarons, a healer and friend. What was most obvious to me as I sat on the side of Gaea's bed was the peace that emanated from her. Here was a woman waiting to have her heart removed in a few hours, waiting for doctors miles away in another hospital to remove her new heart from the body of a dying man. She was totally present, surrendered.

There, in that room, Gaea was the heart of stillness and love, bathing all who entered in peace, whether they were aware of it or not. I realized that, in just being willing to show up, I was being graced with an incredible gift—a demonstration of surrender to that which is eternally present, pure, and radiant self.

I watched Gaea interact with doctors, nurses, attendants, family, and visitors. In all interactions, regardless of the nature of their relationship to her, her relationship to them was the same, as love. She was patient, open, and compassionate, embracing each of them with her peace. It was clear that, instead of people coming to give her assurance in the face of what was to come, she, having already fully met the worst her mind could conjure forth in fear and imagination, was transmitting peace to those who came to her side. What I saw most clearly was that this peace and compassionate love were independent of circumstance.

Here, in the midst of potentially terrifying circumstances, where fear and doubt had every opportunity to arise and drag Gaea's consciousness into all sorts of hell realms, was something hell itself could not touch and where heaven resided.

Somehow there was this incredible certainty that everything was okay, in fact perfect. In this perfection it was totally clear that the operation would be one hundred percent successful. This was not coming from wanting or desiring or praying for a *particular outcome. It was much more solid than any of that. I knew this. There was no doubt.*

Our friends Chris and Karen were also at the hospital on transplant night. They own a wedding chapel in Golden, Colorado.

Karen's Report:

> *I remember a busy Sunday at the chapel. The day before, there had been a sudden, intense storm that dumped a couple of feet of snow on Denver. We had five weddings scheduled, only three of which could take place on Saturday. We rescheduled the other two for Sunday. At the end of the day, as we were walking into our house, we heard the phone ringing. It was Chaitanya sounding very solemn. He told me Gaea's heart had arrived and that she was going to be operated on within the hour. I told Chris and we rushed off to the hospital.*

> *I felt a sense of wonder at the enormity of this event, and honored to be part of it. I also braced myself for what I knew would be a long and intense vigil.*

> *When we arrived at the hospital, we couldn't find Gaea. We went in and out of elevators to various floors and wings, but we kept winding up in the wrong place. After about fifteen minutes of roaming around, we finally found Barry, Sara, and other friends, only to be told that Gaea had just been wheeled away. We were very disappointed to have missed seeing her before the surgery.*

> *We then settled in with everyone in the waiting area. I remember a lot of meditation and prayer, but mostly I remember Sara. We were all very attentive to her. I didn't have to imagine what she was going through—I knew. There were so many times as a child when I had to face the possible loss of my own mother, and I felt very connected to Sara in her fear. Even though I'm not usually very natural or comfortable with children, I found myself holding her hand and just being with her.*

The atmosphere in the semi-darkened waiting area was charged with a mixture of peace, anxiety, guardian angels, and profound community. We were all facing the unknown together. I felt privileged to be witness to this and humbled by the ultimate mystery of life and death. I knew the others were having cosmic visions or whatever in their meditations, and I felt very inept at prayer. All I could do was hold Sara's hand. Eventually, she slept.

Another family sat near us in the waiting area. A loved one was undergoing some kind of multiple transplant. I felt the weight of their anxiety and the vulnerability of us all. I also found myself thinking a lot about the tragedy that had made this new life for Gaea possible—the death of a fifteen-year-old boy. I thought of his family and the unspeakable generosity they had managed to extend to a stranger at such a time.

After some hours, we heard that the surgery was over. All had gone well and we would soon see Gaea wheeled down the hallway across from where we were sitting. It was amazing to see her even for that instant, knowing that a new heart was now beating inside her. I also knew how tentative this all was, that anything, many things, could go awry. But somehow I knew that all would be well. Chris and I went home. I was filled with awe at the magnitude of what had just occurred and felt very grateful to have been present.

Chris' Report:

I'll never forget the time I spent at the hospital with Gaea's dearest friends and family the night she had her heart transplant. Though we just missed seeing her as she was rolled into the operating room, we settled in for the night in a large waiting room. I had never seen Barry's heart so wide open. Karen settled in with Sara, helping her through a very scary night. Gaea's friends included several healers and meditators, and so I felt very comfortable slipping into meditation and healing circles with them.

Our mutual love for Gaea must have intensified our sensitivities because we were all having amazing experiences. I, for one, remember falling into a very deep state where I felt I was standing right next to Gaea and holding her right hand for at least twenty minutes. When her old heart was removed I felt her whole body go into a kind of pure, physical grief. The parting, the separation of the heart from the body, was felt in every cell of her—and my—body, even though she was anesthetized.

Then the experience became even deeper. After a few minutes, the physical sensations of grief faded away, and it seemed that Gaea was in a place where neither life nor death had any meaning. It was not a frightening place at all—actually, it was a place of profound peace, that eternally still center of all being. No longer was I sitting beside her, holding her hand; we were together in this same center.

Mysteriously, I also felt my own hopes and prayers that Gaea would come through the surgery. No conflict existed between the eternal stillness and these prayers and hopes and fears. I felt an incredible sense of community with the doctors and nurses who were tending to Gaea's physical needs, and with her friends and family whose prayers and stillness surrounded her. Together with the doctors, we were all carrying her across this threshold of one heart to another because for these few hours Gaea could not possibly carry herself.

When her new heart was put in, I was at her side again, holding her hand, feeling a new wave of grief from the heart which was taken from a boy who died way too young. Another few minutes of surrender and this grief, too, was discharged into the vastness around us. Perhaps all of this was my own imagination—who can say? But I sensed that Gaea had a capacity for surrender I had not imagined before.

When I returned from my meditations, we found out the operation had been a success, and we all eagerly awaited a chance to see her wheeled from the operating room to ICU. I saw her through a distant glass for one brief moment, and then the long night was over.

Fifteen months after my transplant, I met Laura Roiger, one of the nurses who cared for my donor at the end of his life. This is her report of the night he died.

Laura's Report:

> This story began in the Surgical Intensive Care unit at St. Anthony Hospital. With a snowstorm raging outside, it was impossible for most of us to get home and we slept at the hospital so we could work the next day. Everyone knows it's difficult to sleep in the hospital and I can testify to this truth. My assignment was to care for a young fifteen-year-old boy who had sustained a severe head injury after being hit by a SUV while walking home from a video store. I was soon to learn that because of the injury to his brain he was no longer living and the ventilator was maintaining his body.

> His mother and father were at his bedside trying to understand how it could be that this vibrant teenager wasn't living. After all, his heart was beating; he was warm; and his color was pink. Maybe he was just "sleeping," and if we all wished and prayed hard enough he would wake up and say, "Hi." At times they thought this was a dream and they would wake up and discover it was just a terrible nightmare. Eventually they began to realize that he was not going to wake up and they weren't having a nightmare: they were living the nightmare.

> I witnessed them as gentle and loving and, in the midst of their grief, good and comforting to one another. When the time seemed appropriate, they were approached with an offer to donate his organs and tissues. They were told the miracle they were praying for could happen not for them but for others and that his lasting gift would be his biggest gift of all—giving life to another. They agreed rather quickly to make him an organ and tissue donor.

Three

Going Home

Angels work at University Hospital in Denver. They look like people but definitely act like angels. I had the most wonderful care and loving kindness from everyone, starting with the housekeeper whose radiant smile and loving heart lit up my room every time she entered, to all the skilled and caring nurses and attendants.

The doctors were great, too. One of my favorites was a surgeon from the Ukraine whose loving presence modeled to everyone what true doctoring means. One afternoon she came to check on me and ended up staying about forty-five minutes, telling stories about her life in the Ukraine, her mom, and her mom's cooking. In the journal I kept at the hospital, I even have a few of her recipes. She also worked in the Denver General Hospital emergency room. It was sorrowful work for her, treating many young people with knife and gun wounds whom she felt had no sense of the value of life; she said most of them were in a hurry to get out of the hospital so that they could continue their violent lifestyle. She left Denver at the end of the year and had a job waiting for her in Salt Lake City. Lucky Utah.

I was ecstatic. To be so alive, to feel such strength in my voice (the rest of the body would catch up), was new and thrilling. Barry's brother Neil came to lend support. It meant the world to both of us. Now when people called or visited, I could remember and be present. I laughed a lot, simply feeling the miracle of my new life.

I know I was carried by all the prayers and loving thoughts of many people, known and unknown to me. I say unknown, because someone I knew would call a friend or relative in another city, and there would be a prayer circle there, too. Before the transplant, Barry went to a meditation retreat once a month. Each time he would come back and report that in meditation he received strong messages that I would get a healthy boy's heart, that masters and angels were surrounding me, and that I would have the very best of outcomes. This is how it was and is.

Being a person with a transplant means that I no longer have the medical condition (cardiomyopathy) that precipitated the need for the transplant. On the other hand, I do have another medical condition called post-transplant. That's how the doctors see it, and it makes sense to me. Enormous vigilance is needed to comply with the medication regime, the hospital visits, biopsies, etc. The side effects from steroids started right away with a herpes outbreak. It had been dormant for many years, but my suppressed immune system caused it to surface. It was to be the first of many uncomfortable and sometimes miserable side effects: frequent headaches, swollen face (the full moon look), sore mouth with fungal growth, mental confusion, memory loss, changes in vision, joint and muscle pain, emotional highs, depression, hair loss on my head, hair growth on my face, arms, and legs, sensitivity to cold food—the list goes on. I can laugh about it now because over time, as the dosages of steroids have tapered, the side effects diminished. Even when the various side effects were at their worst, I would remind myself that I was alive to complain, and that was the blessing.

My first biopsy at the hospital showed zero rejection—the greatest news! But my heart was beating too slowly, and the doctors were concerned. I couldn't leave until my heart rate increased.

In the meantime, I started cardiac rehabilitation. I did leg and lung exercises, and I took my first walks down the hall. My legs were so de-conditioned from the time in ICU and the new medications that it was hard going at first. But it was a thrill.

I got my hair washed with the help of a nurse and Barry. It felt so good to be clean. That afternoon, two friends came down to visit. One painted my toenails ruby red; the other took photographs of Barry and me grinning in ecstasy. I felt like a queen!

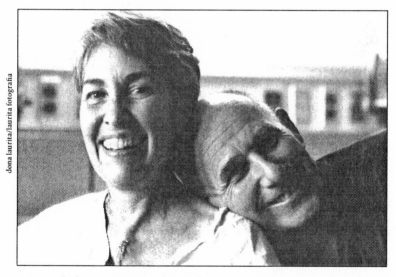

dona laurita/laurita fotografia

I needed a potassium drip. This is a very painful IV that takes hours. I begged them to just give me tons of oral potassium, but it had to be the drip. So I got my tape player, put on headphones, cranked up the volume, played Bach and Mozart, and got through it.

Sunday morning I found myself watching Christian programming on television. Being Jewish by birth and non-denominationally spiritual by nature, this was not my normal style by any stretch of the imagination. Suddenly, I was crying. It occurred to me that my donor was probably Christian, and that while his parents were possibly grieving in church morning, I was in a hospital bed celebrating my new heart and grieving with them.

When my heart started pacing normally the pacemaker wires were removed. Sutures were also removed, but the metal staples up and down my chest from below my throat to the bottom of my sternum would remain for another three weeks.

I received nutritional counseling and instructions about the fifteen or so medications I would be taking home with me, along with the news that I would be going home the next day. This was just four days after leaving the ICU.

Going home the ninth day after surgery? I was scared. I liked knowing that a nurse was down the hall and that my heart telemetry monitors would notify the doctors of any problems. The thought of leaving was frightening. On the other hand, I knew that germs thrive in hospitals, and home would be cleaner and quieter. If the doctors felt I was ready to go, then I needed to trust them. I went home with a huge shopping bag of medications. The doctors said to call the transplant coordinators with any questions, day or night. I have only the fondest memories for the wonderful and loving care I received on the transplant ward at University Hospital.

The drive home was surreal. Everyone and everything moved so fast, I felt as if I was in an altered state. I was euphoric, both from the high dosage of steroids in my system and from the enormity of grace spilling over me with this new heart.

Our house was sparkling, thanks to Barry's all-night cleaning spree. Everything shined from ceiling to floor. Twenty minutes after we arrived home, a new king-size bed was delivered, a welcome-home present from my honey. Twenty minutes after that, Sara walked in the door. I was sitting in the living room waiting for her. What joy on her face to see her mom at home, alive and healthy. This was a celebration for all of us.

Support came from many places, known and unknown. I had no idea what would happen if I simply allowed myself to accept the abundant generosity that was coming my way. There were many times when someone would offer something and my habit would be to say, "Oh no, don't bother," then I caught myself and said "yes." I see now that they were gifted by this. Countless people have thanked me for allowing them to participate in this process, often telling me their lives changed because of it. People held prayer circles and sweat lodges. A client of Barry's lit a candle for me in Notre Dame Cathedral in Paris. The outpouring of support spoke to the open heart everywhere that yearns to be a part of community, to serve. What beauty.

The phone tree that had notified so many friends of my trip to the hospital nine days ago was re-activated with this latest good news, and the gifts of healthy meals that were to sustain us for the next month started to arrive. Was this a community transplant? Absolutely. So many were eager to share in our joy, eager to help in any way possible. Many lives were enriched and, in some cases, changed by it all.

Every day, every moment, was a new frontier. I lost all my guidelines. There were no road maps for this journey. I listened to my body. Energy to write? Did it. Needed to rest? Did it. Very basic, very simple. And always, radiance. My old heart was at the end. The doctors said it had ridges like a prune or a hand that's been in water for twelve hours. No muscle, yellow. I felt I was fading, I said I was fading, but after surgery I understood it in a new way. Friends said they saw my life force draining away more and more each time they saw me, especially the last few months. Now, every cell of my body was being nourished with life force and oxygen for the first time in years. I was so excited! Thank God for my strength of spirit, for my surrender to the limitations of how much "doing" was possible, for my devoted friends and family, and for my willingness to adhere to a rigid no-salt diet. It kept me alive until a heart was available.

The transplant team wanted me to start cardiac rehabilitation five days after I came home. I couldn't believe that they expected me to actually be on treadmills and stationary bikes so soon. I was exhausted from the surgery. But they said, "Yes, come, it's important to start rehabilitation right away." The list of people who could drive me to the hospital for rehab was activated. It was all organized by one friend who called me at the end of each week to tell me who would drive me the next week. This was a great way to spend time with friends because it was a forty-five-minute drive each way. They loved it too.

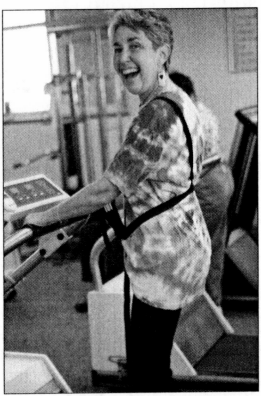

Exercise was my first "new frontier." When I was sick with heart failure, fatigue was a signal to stop and rest. My life depended on it. Many times in the months following surgery I had to push myself. I would tell myself: *Now Gaea, you have a new heart. It loves to move and be active. Your old heart couldn't be active without doing damage to itself and risking your life. Tired does not mean stop like it used to. Normal people get energy from exercise, not to mention the endorphins that kick in. It's okay to exercise when you are tired, in fact it's good for*

you, and you probably won't be so tired afterwards. So I discovered the joy of working out even when I felt resistance and the energy and pride that came with it.

Another new frontier: food. Such total joy! For all my years with heart failure, when I had severely restricted my salt intake, I had avoided restaurants because they prepared food with too much salt. Now I could eat anywhere I wanted. Barry and I stunned everyone we knew by leaving a message on our voice mail the day after I arrived home. "Hi, this is Gaea. I'm home from the hospital! I'm doing great! Tonight Barry and I are going out for Chinese dinner. This will be the first time in six years that I can have Chinese food. Leave a message."

I rested all that day in order to have the energy to go out to eat. Given all the possibilities of restaurants in our town, Chinese was my immediate and gleeful choice. We went to a wonderful place with fresh and tasty food. Every morsel was delectable. I was in heaven and told Barry that if I died right then and there, I would have died happy.

I could eat bagels and store-bought bread for the first time in six years; basically, I could eat anything I wanted. But a transplanted heart is at risk of hardening of the arteries. Knowing that, I began eating a heart-healthy diet of low fat, low cholesterol, and low salt. Occasionally, on special celebrations, I splurge like the rest of humanity, and eat something sinfully rich. Why not? I got a transplant to live, and live I do!

Viewing my wild ride with the many side effects as a new frontier helped me keep a perspective of the enormous challenges I faced. My friend Lerita, who had a heart transplant three years before mine, reminded me that my body was in chaos trying to adjust to the new medications and that this would ease with time. It helped to know this, especially on the hardest days.

In November, just a few weeks after my transplant, I received an excited call from my friend Karin. She had obituaries and information about my donor. I yelled for her to stop before she said anything else. I knew without a doubt that I did not want this information. It was too soon. I couldn't completely explain it, but I was very certain. We ended our conversation quickly. Later, I had a chance to consider what was going on for me about this.

I wasn't ready for information about my donor. I knew that at some point I would be ready and I would feel a resounding "yes" when that time came. I felt there was something operating here in the spirit realm; there would be divine timing.

Karin called a few days later to say she would keep the information for another time, if and when I wanted it. I asked her not to share it with anyone else, especially Barry. I was afraid he'd drop hints if he knew, and I was fiercely holding to my desire to know nothing. She said she would keep the information private for as long as I needed it that way.

I heard a lot about people who took on characteristics of their donors. One heart recipient wrote a book about it. I was skeptical, but if it were a possibility, I wanted to feel it from within. In other words, I wanted no information about my donor. If I was to experience any aspect of him, I didn't want known facts to influence me.

There was another reason. I felt compassion for my donor's family and all that they went through. Out of respect, I didn't want to know anything about him or them before they wanted me to. I would wait.

But Barry had to know. He promised he would give absolutely no hint of anything he learned. He got the information and kept his promise. He never raised an eyebrow or gave any information away. Every once in a while he would check in with me about this again: Was I really sure I didn't want to know anything? My answer was always the same. I wasn't ready, and I would know when the time was right.

By December, six weeks after surgery, I was starting to feel shut down, in a rut. The problem was that I only allowed myself to feel gratitude, and there was a lot more going on. Holding on to "only gratitude" was making me false to myself, and I got depressed. In truth, the gratitude didn't diminish when I admitted I was uncomfortable. I could feel both the gratitude and the discomfort at the same time, which was more authentic.

When I tried to keep discomfort at bay, I stopped thinking about my donor and his family, and I shut down. When I allowed myself to feel everything, I opened again to a depth of gratitude to my donor's family, my gift of life.

Seven weeks after my transplant, I was euphoric when the three of us went for a two-and-a-half-hour hike! Barry and Sara watched me in amazement as we went up some pretty steep hills. When we came home, they joined me in writing letters to my donor's family. We sent them to Donor Alliance, the organ procurement agency, and they forwarded the letters to the family. I loved Sara's letter and saved a copy.

Dear Family,   12-14-97

Thanks, for letting your son's heart become my mothers. Its like sharing one heart together. Now that my mom has a new heart she can do some more things. If your son didn't give his heart up well my mother probily wouldn't have lived.

This is a picture of my mom.

Love
Sarah R Shaw

My log
TARA   Dad   MOM   Me

Christmas was coming soon, and so was the two-month anniversary of my transplant. My dear heart was heavy, grieving many losses—my mother, my father, my sister, and so many others, and I knew that my donor's family must have been feeling immense grief at this time of the year. It was such a contrast, to have my life again, yet to feel the grief so strongly.

Melanie encouraged me to create some sort of ritual of acknowledgement and to do it soon. I decided to light sixteen large red candles—one for myself, the others for my donor. Sitting quietly, I felt his spirit in the room with me. I had a vision of a boy with short blond hair, wearing a shirt and gray pullover sweater. He was smiling and at peace. When I told Barry about it, he had a strong sense that my donor's name was Kevin. Peter is what came to me.

Before the surgery my friend Lerita said there would be a time when "courageous" would fit me. By January, I knew what she meant. I was laid low by the side effects of the medications. I felt drugged, in a mental fog, spacey, shaky. My mouth was numb, and something was going on with my gums because anything cold in my mouth hurt. My face and hands were swollen; my eyes were puffy. My legs, knees, and ankles were weak. All this was experienced right along side the incredible gift of a new heart, new life.

I yearned for quiet. There was much to integrate. There was nothing I needed to do except to be sure I didn't get too busy. With Sara home from school for winter break, there wasn't much time for quiet and solitude. I was challenged by exercise, because my ankles and knees hurt when I worked out vigorously. I decided to try my luck at swimming because it would be a gentler form of working out. Except for an occasional dip and splash, I hadn't been in a pool since I was a child.

I was due for another biopsy and I prayed for another zero so I could cut back on the steroids a little, which would decrease the side effects. I didn't accomplish much. I needed lots of rest. I wondered if anesthesia was lingering in my system.

On my third-month anniversary, I wrote this in my journal:

> *Beloved Heart, beloved soul who gave your heart to me, I am so blessed, even in the midst of discomfort with a cold and aching muscles. I want to live a life worthy of this gift. Can I?*

Will I? What does that mean? I know it is about living fully, yet isn't that what all beings must strive for? Perhaps the gift is to see so strongly, and feel such gratitude, for every breath and every new day here, alive, with family and friends, and sky and trees and birds and dogs and cats and mountains. On and on!

Last week, I swam—good medicine for me! The water was calming and nurturing. Being immersed in the slightly warm water soothed this body, agitated by my medication's side effects. I was excited to make it across the pool more than once. I was relieved to find exercise that didn't hurt. Before that, I had injured myself on a rowing machine. I'm beginning to get the picture: This body is not used to exertion. The heart is ready, yes, but muscles and joints need ease and gentle entry into the world of exercise.

What a blessing and what a challenge! It is possible to feel both at once. Because it's all here. This body is going through it! I am zapped, wiped out, humbled by this journey. The doctors are right; recovery takes about a year. With only three months behind me, I have a long way to go.

Am I grateful? Absolutely! For a beautiful sunrise, for being alive, for the courage to take this journey, for the loving support of family and friends, for spirit's presence in my life.

Our gift fund allows me these months to recover and not return to work. What a blessing! I am being carried by so many people! And Barry, working extra hard and long hours to take care of us. I'm glad he's taking the day off today. He needs the rest.

A few days later it was Sara's tenth birthday. She was full of glee, radiating joy, but I was sick, so Barry handled Sara's party. He helped her decorate, did all the shopping, and took six girls bowling. What a guy! Always caring, devoted, a constant source of love. I am incredibly lucky to have such a beautiful man in my life.

I stayed in bed. Being sick didn't diminish my deep sense of gratitude. It was a beautiful, glorious day. The windows were open wide to let in the fresh air. The house was quiet and I rested, allowing my body to repair itself.

Sara is one of my reasons for the transplant—knowing my work as a parent wasn't finished, that she needed me in her life. I hoped then, as I do now, that I would be around to see the big milestones: high school graduation, college if she wants it, marriage, as well as the joy of being here to experience each day and the small, seemingly trivial moments. After such a life-changing event, even little things can feel significant.

I was on a roller-coaster ride. Two weeks after Sara's birthday, I asked Barry if he thought I was depressed. He laughed and said, "No, you're not depressed, you've just been through hell." That helped put it all in perspective.

By March 1998 I was well over my cold and had the energy to swim and walk. It was a thrill to feel so much life force.

March 13, 1998

> *I swam laps for forty minutes on Wednesday. Yahoo! The gift of life, of this heart, is beyond words. I am so filled with gratitude. In people's deepest grief, to agree to allow their loved one's organs to be donated—well, it's incredible, beyond any words. Today I am exuberant and joyous, filled with immense gratitude, love.*

March 17, 1998

> *"I'm so sorry." These words come as a powerful jolt tonight. Guilt that I'm having so much fun and feeling so good. Some ancient message that there should be a cap to my joy.*
>
> *Everyone is so busy, working hard, exhausted; and I have this freedom of free time to swim, walk, play . . . some strong sense that it is not okay to have this much fun. These thoughts could undermine my forward progress. I'm alarmed.*

A few days after my journal entry about guilt, it was time for a biopsy. I was on top of the world, swimming, hiking, and riding my bike. I told the doctor I didn't really need a biopsy; after all, I was active and feeling great.

The next day the rug was pulled out from under me when the nurse called to say that I was in rejection. I was devastated. If there was any corner of my mind where I had become complacent or took things for granted, it was slapped out of me then and there. I was humbled and shaken to the core. The rejection would have made more sense to me if I were feeling rotten. How could this be? Maybe they mixed up my results with somebody else's. No, they explained, the probable explanation for rejection when I was feeling so good was that they caught it in the early stages. Had the biopsy been a month later, I most likely would have felt the signs, such as exhaustion and shortness of breath.

There is an antidote for rejection, and I started on "the drill" right away. My steroid dosage went up to almost twenty times more than I had been taking. I went from 7 1/2 milligrams of prednisone a day to 120 milligrams. The other steroids went up too. It was an enormous blast, and it worked. A week later, I was out of rejection but still on high doses of steroids. There was a short period of steroid-induced euphoria, and then I entered "the hell realm," dropping into a world of utter misery. I was flattened; my world was in chaos. The drugs caused this. I was disorganized internally; time passed with no sense of time. I actually felt psychotic. I'd be comatose one moment and edgy the next. My eating was out of control; I had insomnia; my knees and ankles started hurting again; my face swelled up; and I had frequent throbbing headaches. I have spoken to other transplant recipients who have had rejection episodes, and they also experienced many of the same miserable symptoms from the high steroid dosages.

Barry helped me by reminding me more than once that this was a chemically induced state. I don't know how he and Sara put up with me. One morning I awakened, leaned over to cuddle with Barry and told him that I wanted my old heart back. What a shock! I can honestly say that it was the only time when I wondered if getting a transplant was worth it.

I felt vulnerable, young, and needed to stay safe for a while. I couldn't watch any violence on TV, didn't go out a lot, stayed quiet, and didn't socialize. I had some long-distance healings from Melanie. I asked for quiet in the house, laid down in bed, and Melanie sent me healing energy from her house. Those sessions helped ground me and keep me a bit more sane. Even in the depths of despair from this drug-induced state, there was occasional recognition of the grace and blessings that never went anywhere.

April 6, 1998

What a ride. Yesterday the dark cloud lifted. I knew the minute I awoke. Barry and I went for a four-and-a-half-mile hike. It felt great. The doom and gloom of the past week is gone.

Today I am tired (awoke at 4:00 a.m.) and have a busy day, with early hospital lab work, driving Sara to gymnastics, and shopping for groceries. This might seem like nothing to the average person, but for me it's a lot. I nicknamed my experience of side effects from prednisone the "predni-zone." When I'm in the "predni-zone," one activity a day is enough. I get overwhelmed quite easily.

April 8, 1998

Still so much body stuff—headaches, throbbing in my head and ears, buzzing and tingling, aching ankles and knees, discomfort in my mouth, sensitivity to cold, and other weird sensations.

Yet I have some sense of having turned the corner with the "predni-zone." A returning groundedness and predictability. "If I do too much, then I will feel overwhelmed." A sense of returning order.

I had another "visit" from my donor's spirit. It came during a session with Melanie. I got a message that he was confused, feeling "all in pieces," very vulnerable. He needed comfort and reassurance, as if to say, "Okay, I have been here for you, now I need you to be here for me." I called my friend Karin, half-

crazed and not knowing what to do. She suggested I get very quiet and take my donor there with me to that quiet.

I did. We are very peaceful. He likes this. This is how I can be here for him. I am not accustomed to getting or feeling messages from spirit, but I trust this one hundred percent.

I'm feeling fragile, even though I also feel robust strength. I'm very tired, not getting much sleep.

April 10, 1998

I went for an early morning swim after a good long sleep. I feel wonderful! Today has been a day of sudden connections, and I have shed many tears of fullness, not sadness. I met a woman whose mom had a liver transplant seven years ago. As she told her story, we both cried. A woman in the grocery store asked me about my transplant T-shirt that read, "I got a new life at the University Hospital Transplant Center." "Is it true?" "Yes." "What?" "Heart." I hugged and cried with this woman I had never met. Later in the day I shared with Barry about the seedling awareness of my donor, and the tears flowed again.

April 12, 1998

Whew. I was blasted by a nine-hour migraine yesterday. The pain was intense; I couldn't handle light or sound and could barely talk. Because of the medications I take, I can't have the normal painkillers that other people take for migraines. I had to go to the ER to get shots of Demerol for the pain and Compasine for the nausea. I waited four hours to see a doctor. It was hell. Barry was on the edge, feeling helpless, and Sara needed reassurance that my life was not in danger. Today I am much better, calm, quiet, and eating simply.

I am afraid of being in rejection again. I have a biopsy in three days. I will not ignore this fear; instead, I will bring it to the quiet and be with it. I love my new dear heart that brings *me renewed life force and vibrancy. Everything, highs and lows, comes to the new aliveness that is here for me.*

April 15, 1998

Zero rejection! Whoopee! I am so lucky! A vibrant new heart, surrounded by so much love, grace, beauty. My heart is strong, and I feel so good after exercise. Today I hiked a few miles—it was a fast-paced, strenuous hike. What a great feeling. I love feeling my heart beating steadily, strongly. Ah, the blessings, the challenges.

May 6, 1998

I worry that I am in rejection again or that something else is wrong with me—skin cancer, brain damage, high cholesterol, that I'll need another heart. These mind-spins come and go. Add to that, guilt: if I have those thoughts, I must be ungrateful. Oh, how hard I am on myself. No mercy.

Today I will strive to be loving and compassionate toward myself, one moment at a time.

Three weeks after these journal entries, the dosage of one of my steroids was lowered a bit, and I started feeling more normal and rosy. The drugs really played havoc physically, mentally, and emotionally. Then I experienced peace at my core, and I saw how grace, peace, and love surround and underline my daily life. Events agitate only superficially. In a healing session with Melanie, she saw my guides, my beaming donor, and his guides. I have many angels watching over me—I have a double set!

Four

1998

Back in March, even though I was dealing with rejection, I had called the Denver chapter of the National Kidney Foundation to inquire about the Olympic-style U.S. Transplant Games that they organize and present. Every other year, people of all ages, with all kinds of life-saving transplants, gather to participate and compete in a variety of athletic events. Knowing I wasn't an accomplished athlete, I couldn't imagine going. I was assured that the level of skill went from couch potato to elite athlete, and that all transplant recipients were welcome to participate if their doctors gave them permission. What I learned got me very excited.

The NKF sent a ten-minute video about the 1996 games in Utah for me to view. I had never seen so many recipients at once, all going "full out" to do the best with their new lives. I was hooked. I sobbed through the entire video. I had to go, and I wanted Barry and Sara to go. They had been through so much; I knew this would be a celebration for all of us. I showed them the video and they were hooked, too.

One way or another, we would find the financial resources to make that trip.

The games would be held in early August in Columbus, Ohio. I was such a rookie in the arena of athletics that when the application for the games asked for the name of the competitor, I didn't know what it meant. Surely it couldn't be me! I had a good laugh about that! I had never competed athletically in my entire life. Boy, was I scared. Then I had another good laugh. After all I had been through, facing death and a transplant, I was scared about competing in some games.

"The competitor" was being born and I had no time to lose. Since I loved swimming so much, it would be my event at the games. I started training with a vengeance. The only problem was that I hadn't taken lessons in fifty years. My form was lousy; my times were pitiful. I became friends with Liz Kaplan, the head swimming instructor at our local recreation center. Liz started to help me with my swim stroke and became very excited that I was going to Columbus. With that was birthed the next wonderful opportunity.

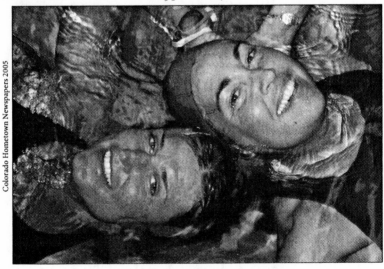

In the pool, Liz and me

I went to our local city council and requested free swimming practice and free coaching with Liz in preparation for the games. They cheerfully granted it, wished me well, and asked me to return after the games to report how they went for me.

Liz and I were off and running. She's a great coach, and I learned how to swim all over again. I remember one turn-around conversation, when I told Liz that I wanted to compete but didn't care if I won or not. She gave me a look as only a coach can and said, "Now, Gaea, as long as you're going, why not win!" This was all new territory for me: training, timing myself, pushing myself. I absolutely loved it. I was exhausted and sore from the hard work. And I was proud.

It was the end of May. My last biopsy was a zero (the best news!); my swimming was awesome; my times were getting better; and I was filled with gratitude for this dear heart that was making all of this possible. Lab tests showed I needed more steroids to keep my heart from rejecting, and I hoped for no major side effects. I got shaky hands, swollen eyes, and other uncomfortable but bearable sensations. Swimming helped. When I got in the water my body was more at ease.

I swam as much as a half mile four or five days a week. For this woman who couldn't swim one length of the pool a year ago, it was magical and magnificent, truly awesome. I was constantly aware of the blessings and of the gratitude I felt toward the donor family I had never met, who had given me this second chance at life.

Training continued in earnest. In June I sent a letter to one hundred people asking for donations in my name to the National Kidney Foundation. By then I knew that most people want to serve and help; all they need is to know what to do. I had no problem asking for support because I understood this so well. The contributions poured in. Because there was such a strong response to my letter, the National Kidney Foundation was able to give us some financial assistance. To our delight, Coach Liz was able to go, too, because an anonymous donor paid her way.

I seem to belong to the "never a dull moment" club of life. On July 2, my birthday, I was driving our little car and was rear-ended by a big truck whose driver said the brakes locked and he couldn't stop. I had no visible bruises or broken bones, and my blessed heart was fine. But my neck, back, ribs, and shoulders were all very sore, and I began to get frequent headaches. I faced the probability that I wouldn't be able to go to the games or, if I went, I wouldn't be at my best.

Then, good old grace and grit kicked in, and I decided that, win, lose, or draw, I was going. I went to one or another type of physical therapy at least three times a week, absolutely determined to do whatever I could to get my body back into shape. One month later, we were all on the plane to Columbus, Ohio.

Every state had a team at the games. Team Colorado had thirty-nine athletes, ranging in age from eighteen months to sixty-nine years. There were fifteen kidney, ten lung, six liver, five heart, one heart-double lung, and two bone marrow recipients. Along with family-support members and five donor families, there were about seventy people on the team. The two youngest members, a toddler and a four year old, were both heart recipients. They participated in children's track and field events. They were precious.

It's challenging to find words to describe such an inspiring event. In all, there were fifteen hundred athletes (transplant recipients) and six hundred donor-family members. This was the first time that a gathering of donor-family members that large was combined with the games. We all wore color-coded nametags, so when we walked around we could tell who was a recipient, family-support member, living donor (i.e., kidney donor), or donor-family member.

The opening ceremonies were held in the stadium at the Ohio State University. Each team entered as a group, in the style of the Olympics, and carried a banner naming their state. I cried or laughed all week from the inspiration and joy that I felt, being in the company of so many brave souls. That evening, walking into the stadium with Team Colorado, I wept. At the other end of the stadium were thousands of cheering family-support members and donor-family members, honoring all of us who had been through so much and who were there to celebrate the victory of our second chance at life. How could I be so lucky? It was a thrill, an extraordinary feeling! After a touching ceremony honoring all the donor families that were present, and then too many speeches, the Olympic-style torch was lit and the games officially began.

The next few days were devoted to the athletic events. I kept looking around, realizing that each of the fifteen hundred participants would not be alive to compete at the games if it weren't for the gift of life they'd been blessed with. I had ample opportunity to thank the many donor-family members I met.

The competitive events were awesome. The athletes came in all shapes and sizes with varying degrees of ability. Some were blind, some were on oxygen. Some needed a cane or a wheelchair. One young man had no legs from the knees down or arms below the elbows, but that didn't stop him from competing. Everyone was there to celebrate life and to show the world what's possible after a transplant. Those who needed help to cross the finish line and those who came in last received the loudest cheers for their courage, effort, and perseverance.

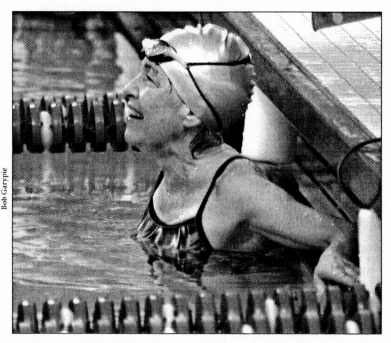

Bob Garypie

My swimming events were on the last day. During training sessions, Liz had prepared me for the hundreds of people who would be watching and cheering, and for the five swimmers who would line up next to me on the diving blocks. She had even held my hand the first few times I used a diving block because I was scared. Then, there I was in Columbus, not really scared any more but very excited. I absolutely loved racing. I would have done each race two or three times if I could have. It was over way too soon.

I swam the fifty-meter freestyle and won the gold! I swam the five-hundred-meter freestyle and won the gold again! I swam the fifty-meter backstroke and won the silver! Within seconds of the first win, I was profoundly struck by the realization that my greatest joy was not in winning the medals but in being alive, being there, and being able to compete full out. That was the true victory. In my mind, every participant at the games was a gold medal winner. To this day, that is how I see it.

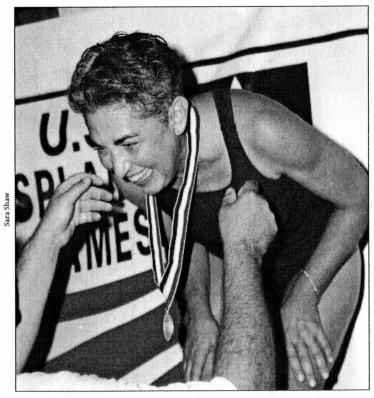

1998, U.S. Transplant Games, receiving my first gold medal

Two unforgettable memories linger from the pool that day. The first occurred when it was announced that a young man winning a bronze medal would receive that medal from the mother of his organ donor, and this was their first meeting. I watched as she put the ribbon around his neck. They hugged tearfully, holding each other for a long time. Then he took off his medal and placed it around her neck. I treasure the photo I have of that moment.

The second unforgettable memory was when the young man with only stumps for arms and legs swam the length of the pool. He used the lane closest to the ledge, and whenever he needed to stop and rest, he put his upper arm on the ledge, took a breath, and then continued. Time seemed to stop as we all stood to watch. I can still feel that moment in my body. Everyone was weeping and crying and cheering as he finished the race. In the face of enormous challenge, he showed so much determination, such fierce resolve. The inspiration of those days in Columbus reached its peak for me at that moment.

Barry and Sara were profoundly moved. When I won the first gold medal, Barry hugged me. We sobbed in recognition of what we had been through to come to that moment. During the closing ceremonies, Sara reached over to her daddy for a hug and thanked him for all his love and support through the last year. What a victory, what a celebration of our family's courage and faith.

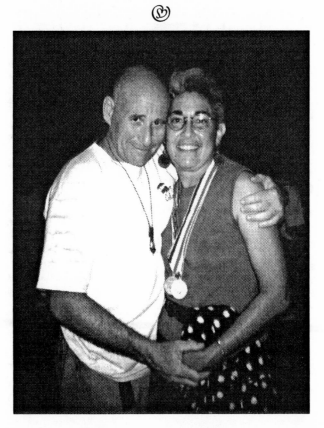

The games were such a high, each moment so inspiring, that I didn't know what to do with myself when I came home. My focus had been strong and clear for months, and now it was over. I was at a loss. I yearned to be with the new and wonderful friends I met in Columbus. I wasn't alone. My new transplant buddies reported the same feelings. It seemed to take all of us a few weeks to land and re-enter our present reality. Everyone was already anticipating meeting at the next games.

With the next U.S. games two years away, swimming took on a different light. Liz encouraged me to keep up my practices, but the motivation was missing. However, I knew I needed the exercise and I wanted to honor my new heart, so I started swimming again. In September I started writing this story and volunteered to speak for Donor Alliance, the organization in Denver that handles organ procurement. I shared my story with any group that wanted to hear about my transplant.

A few months after returning from Columbus, I celebrated the first anniversary with my new heart. The day was quiet, filled with a mix of thoughts and emotions. I knew that I most likely wouldn't be alive if it weren't for the transplant. The surgery and following seven or eight months had been a blessed, holy ordeal. My anniversary was just blessed and holy. I thought of my donor and his family, wondering if they started to find any peace around their loss. I sent them prayers and hoped they would receive them. I already understood that the best way to express my gratitude was to live life fully and appreciate the blessing of each day.

I thought about how much Barry had done for Sara and me, and how lucky we all were. I was still edgy at times and not easy to be with. It seemed so unfair to Barry. I felt immense gratitude for all that was given me, for all the masters and angels who looked after us so lovingly.

I wrote a second letter to my donor's family. Again it was sent to Donor Alliance and forwarded to the family. I thanked them for their incredible gift and told them how well I was doing, including news of my success at the Transplant Games.

I never doubted I would meet my donor's family someday and that after our meeting we would have a continuing relationship. I expected it would be a long time before we met because I knew that losing a child had to be so painful; I just couldn't imagine that they would be ready to meet us anytime soon.

Two weeks later I got a call from Donor Alliance that my donor's mother had brought gifts for all the recipients of her son's organs and that the family wanted to meet us soon. I was stunned. What gifts could they give me? They had already given me a second chance at life!

I wept after I got the call, as we drove to Donor Alliance, while we were there looking at our gifts, and that night at home. They wanted to meet us! I was finally ready to learn about my donor; I had been waiting for his family to reach out to us.

The gifts turned out to be beautiful photos of my donor, Christopher Kuhlman, his mother, Joni, his father, George, and his brother, Peter. There were stories about and by him and letters from the family to us.

Christopher was a beautiful, talented, bright, loving, fifteen-year-old boy. He was walking home from a video store in his hometown in the mountains when he was hit by a car that lost control on the icy roads. His family was reassured that he felt no pain and had no time to be scared. They were certain that, loving and giving as he was, Christopher would have wanted them to donate his organs. Six people's lives were saved, and his corneas were also donated, giving sight to two people.

His mother wrote in her letter to me that Christopher had a kind, thoughtful, and strong heart. I knew this to be absolutely true, and I knew it before she told me. It's what I felt from this wonderful boy from the first moment. I felt his strength and beauty, and I knew that he had a loving family. I felt it in my heart. Christopher's heart embodies this love and kindness, and in some beautiful and mysterious way, I am blessed with the receiving of that. Joni, Christopher's mother, also wrote that he loved to swim!

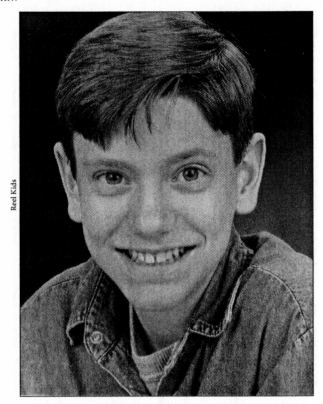

Reel Kids

Christopher Kuhlman, March 14, 1982–October 26, 1997

The gratitude and blessings I had felt every day since my surgery now had a face to it, with a family I would get to meet and thank. I was in awe of how this continued to unfold. I was sure that our meeting each other would help their grief. We were thrilled.

The Kuhlmans chose Valentine's Day 1999 to meet our family, and they wanted the event to be public, to honor their beloved son as a hero. Donor Alliance made the arrangements. We met at Boetcher Mansion in the mountains near Golden, Colorado. There were journalists from three TV stations and two newspapers. The nurses who had cared for Christopher in his final hours were there, too.

It was a day I'll treasure for the rest of my life. After Barry, Sara, and I settled in, the Kuhlmans walked in and the cameras started rolling. Joni called "Gaea!" and came to hug me. She asked if she could hear my heart, and of course I said yes. Everyone was crying, including the journalists and videographers. I presented the Kuhlmans with a heart-shaped wreath made of dried pink roses and one of my gold medals, framed with a plaque in honor of Christopher. Joni was deeply moved by the medal. Christopher is her hero; certainly Christopher and all the Kuhlmans are mine.

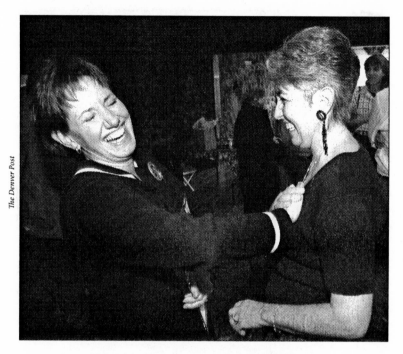

Valentines Day, 1999, meeting Joni Kuhlman

We were all interviewed. What a day! Peter, Christopher's younger brother, was fifteen years old, the age Christopher was when he died. I remembered my vision at Christmas of a young boy standing before me. This was before I knew any details about who he was or who his family was. I had told Barry then that I thought my donor's name was Peter. I was taken aback when I first saw Peter Kuhlman. It was he, not Christopher, who was in my vision. Perhaps Peter came to me so he could be near his brother.

We have ongoing contact with the Kuhlmans. They are beautiful, generous, kind, lovely people. Their grief and loss is immense, of course. But they have told me that donating Christopher's organs gave them a sense of purpose out of the tragedy that was so devastating. They say I'm a living memorial to Christopher. I feel that every day. I send them flowers on Mother's Day and Christopher's birthday. I send them prayers and love whenever I think of them, and I think of them often.

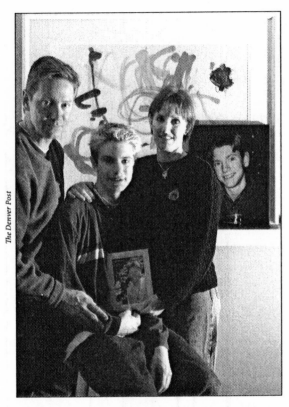

February, 1999, George, Peter, and Joni Kuhlman
with Christopher's photo

Joni and Peter came to the 2000 Transplant competitions in Florida to cheer me on as I swam. I was thrilled and proud that they came, and they were allowed to present me with medals for the events I won. Joni told me it was hard to be there; it intensified her sense of Christopher's loss. I understand.

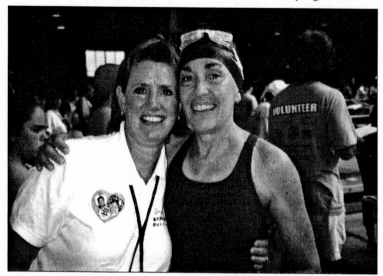

2000 U.S. Transplant Games, at the pool with Joni

I am honored to know the Kuhlmans. I hold the heart that once beat inside their son. When Joni was pregnant with him, it beat inside her. Whew.

Since our first meeting with the Kuhlmans, I have competed in five Transplant Games, including the World Transplant Games in Japan and France, winning a total of twelve gold and six silver medals. I find inspiration and renewed purpose each time I go to the Transplant Games. "Have a transplant, see the world" is my new motto. I absolutely love the opportunity to compete and spend time with other transplant recipients and donor families. God willing and the body able, I'll continue to compete. Ah, the people you meet! The moments you share! It always comes back to this: I am blessed beyond measure.

At the 2004 U.S. Games in Minneapolis, I met many donor family members. One man will always hold a warm place in my heart. When I met him I was already in tears after speaking to his wife. She told me about their son, a young policeman who died from an aneurism while at work. His organs and tissues were donated. When the father learned that I'm a heart recipient, he wrapped his arms around me and wept. Then he told me this story: Shortly after his son's death, an angel came to him in a dream. The angel said his heart was like a shattered glass, and that every time he met an organ recipient the pieces of his shattered heart would mend.

As I look back on what I have written I am struck by two common themes: courage and gratitude. My transplant journey transformed me from a fearful, constricted person to someone who can reach out for the grace and blessings that are always here for me, for you, for *everyone*.

People tend to compare their illnesses and life situations to mine. "I need surgery," or "I've been out of work for a month," they'll say, "but compared to what you went through I have no reason to complain." I discovered courage through my journey, but I have no singular ownership of it. Just to be alive brings its challenges that must be faced. I see courage everywhere.

My grandmother used to say, "If we hung all our friends' problems on a clothesline, then went to pick whose problems we wanted, we'd probably end up choosing our own." Comparisons create suffering. They are endless and fruitless.

Of course there is pain in life and a whole host of situations that could bring on misery and suffering. I am not speaking of denying anything but of experiencing everything completely—and not just with little peeks into the closet of supposed demons.

We can face the inevitable: our own mortality. Once the illusion that we will live forever is shattered, there is the recognition that *there is only this day*—what will *you* make of this day, this moment?

We can recognize and acknowledge our own courage and see where, regardless of circumstances, we can feel grateful. Is it for the sunrise? For our next breath? Suffering simply cannot stick when blessings and grace are so apparent. Take it from a winner who looked death in the face and lived to tell about it.

Epilogue

October 26, 2004

Picky, picky, picky. Yesterday I was swimming—slowly—bemoaning how slow I am. Then I started laughing. What a joke! Here I am, alive and kicking (literally), swimming one thousand yards or more at a time and complaining that I'm not fast enough! How many people my age (sixty-four at this writing) with or without a transplant are swimming a thousand yards once or twice a week, lifting weights twice a week, raising a teenager, working part time, taking long walks, and so on?

Today is the seventh anniversary of my new beloved heart. I will swim a mile today for Christopher. I am honored and humbled by this journey. This gift of life has profoundly affected me, every person in my family, friends, and even strangers.

Sometimes I see my life in terms of what I haven't missed because I'm still here! This past June, Barry and I celebrated our twentieth wedding anniversary, a true testament to our love, devotion, perseverance, and trust through enormous hardship. Things that many people take for granted have special significance for me: seeing Sara go on her first date, helping her choose her first prom dress, teaching her to drive, taking time to smell the roses, and my work as an after-school homework center coordinator at my local library. The list is long and full. Even the smallest event will often have an added twist to it, knowing that the blessing of this new life made it all possible.

On the other hand, I have also experienced some major setbacks. At the end of 1999, two years after my transplant, I was diagnosed with breast cancer. That news struck me harder than when I found out that I needed a transplant. I was devastated and cried for days. Then I put my research skills and my newly acquired habit of asking for support into action. I got a Ph.D. in breast cancer in about two weeks. I got support and information from all corners of this continent, from friends as well as from people I had never met before but who heard my call for help.

So many decisions to make: lumpectomy? mastectomy? radiation?

I didn't need chemo; my cancer was caught early and was non-invasive. I decided against Tamoxifen (a common drug used after cancer but with serious risk factors) because my transplant medications are complicated and I didn't want to add another to the mix. Additionally, with my suppressed immune system, I would have been more likely to experience the drawbacks of Tamoxifen. So, I said no. Strongly. And got no argument from the oncologist.

I fired my first breast cancer surgeon. She was well known and highly respected but I found her heartless, cold, and rushed. My second doctor was more compassionate and took more time with me. I decided to have a lumpectomy and radiation, but the first lumpectomy didn't get the edges of the cancer. I had to have a second surgery, followed by six weeks of radiation. It was grueling. It was painful. I hated it.

The one saving grace during each treatment was visualizing Barry, Sara, or one of my friends with me in the room, holding my hand. I love dolphins, and I visualized them swimming in the ocean of that room and surrounding me with their playful loving energy. The treatment room has a huge radiation machine. I was in the room alone with a six-inch lead door between the technician and me. There was a loud clunking noise when the radiation started. I imagined that the noise was a gate opening and letting the dolphins in and that the noise of the machine was the ocean.

I put the experience behind me and only look back once a year when I have my annual mammogram, a highly charged and nerve-wracking experience for me. But all my mammogram results since then have been clear, so I keep knocking on wood and moving on.

Only months after radiation was completed, in October 2000, my annual exam discovered blocked coronary arteries. Oh my God. This about took me over the top with grief and fear. I had an angioplasty and a stent (a tiny mesh tube inserted in an artery) that very day, a procedure to open the blockage. I have had four annual exams since then. The stent has held up fine, and there has been no further blockage.

Medical challenges continue, but they are interspersed with periods of such abundant health that I almost forget I'm a transplant recipient.

Sara is a junior in high school, thinking about going to college. We have weathered many teenage storms and come out the other side. She's a true delight to be with. I'm proud to be her mama.

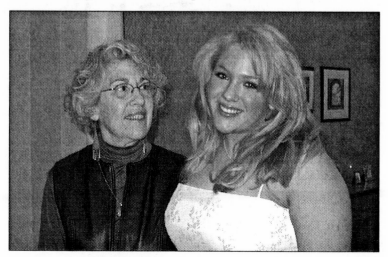

January 2005, Sara is ready for the Winter Ball

Barry, the love of my life, is a jewel. He's devoted to his work and his family. Like me, he feels gratitude every day for this life we have been given. And what a life it is!

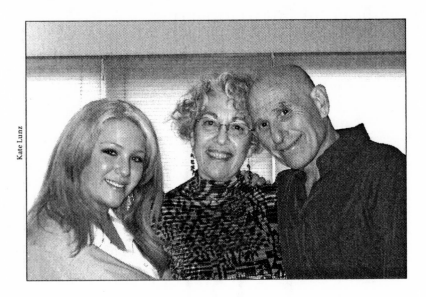

Kate Lunz

Afterword

Before this book was published I asked the Kuhlmans to read it.
Here is a part of their response:

Dear Gaea,

> *Your story is so poignant because as you were together
> celebrating renewed life, we were grieving for our precious lost
> life. We don't remember a lot of things that entire first year,
> especially that horrible night.*

> *The small consolation for us is that our loved one has passed
> his life on to you and so many others who would not be with us
> today if that decision would not have been made.*

Anything to provide donor awareness and how it can take a tragic event to a positive, comforting, and loving experience to all of those who have lost special loved ones is a good thing to promote.

Love,

Joni and George Kuhlman

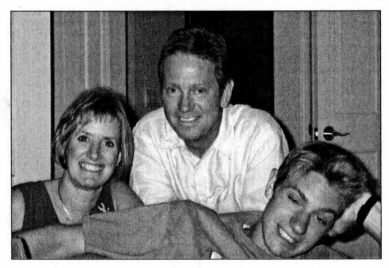

Joni, George, and Peter

Appendix 1

Letters to and from Our Donor Family

We sent cards and letters to our donor family seven weeks after my transplant, long before we met them or knew anything about them. Sara's letter is in the body of this book. Here are the letters that Barry and I wrote, as well as the letters our donor family sent to us a year later.

December 14, 1997

To the Family of my Heart Donor,

Dearest, dearest ones, it is seven weeks today of my living with a new heart donated by your child. You have been in my thoughts and prayers so many times.

I cannot imagine anything more painful than losing a child. It simply is not in the natural order of things for a child to go first. I am the mother of a ten-year-old girl, and I have wept, thinking of you, putting myself in your place.

I want you to know how incredible the gift of this heart has been. For the last six years I lived with a deteriorating heart condition. Medications helped me maintain some semblance of a normal life, but eventually I had to stop working and stop most activity. When I was listed for a transplant, I prayed for a new heart to come soon, because I knew my life force was waning.

In the midst of what I imagine must have been acute and agonizing grief, you found a way to turn the tragedy of your son's death into a gift of life for six people, including me. I hope that, in the midst of all you must be feeling, there is some small comfort in knowing that you helped bring life to all six of us.

This new heart brings much-needed oxygen and vibrant life to every cell and every organ in my body. I have strength and vitality as I have never known. My daughter and husband rejoice at my new energy and life force. I feel so profoundly blessed to have received your son's heart. There are no words to adequately express my gratitude for your decision.

With love and respect and much appreciation,

Gaea Shaw

December 14, 1997

Dear Family,

I am indebted for life for the irony of your son's death that gave my loving wife a new heart and thus a new life.

As a parent of a ten-year-old adopted girl, I sit in total compassion for what your family must be going through. The enormity of life's mysterious challenges are beyond any explanation I've found.

As somebody who is bathed in God's awareness, I can only honor this whole bittersweet process of your son's passing. My wife was close to death with heart failure. We waited for a donor for four months. I knew she was going to get a beautiful vibrant heart of a young boy, and she did.

I want you to know we are sitting in total awe of Gaea's miracle of embodying your son's life. In some way your son's vitality and joy are gracing a whole lot of people.

We mourn your loss. We embrace you for the courage to donate your son's organs in order that people are granted the unbelievable gift supreme—life.

We don't know you but we pray for you. Your son's soul is on the next supreme level we know nothing of. I trust and believe that he is still thriving and playing and laughing and missing you a whole lot.

God be with you always. I'd love to meet you if that's appropriate some day.

> *In Deep Respect,*
>
> *Barry Shaw*

A year later, Christopher's family sent all the recipients of Christopher's organs a packet of letters and photos.

Dearest Recipients,

I hope this letter finds you all well and healthy. I've been meaning to write to all of you for the past year to tell you about Christopher, but I just couldn't do it! Now it's time, with pride and love, to introduce you to the wonderful child who helped you.

First off, Christopher loved life!! He appreciated the beauty of nature and the togetherness of our family. From the minute he was born, we knew he was extremely special. He didn't even cry!! You could tell he was very intelligent, that was my grandmother's first comment. He did all of his firsts very early. He started crawling at five months, walking at nine months, talking and feeding himself at ten months.

Chris was very independent and determined! He was in gifted programs K-8, then in honors classes in high school. One of his favorite pastimes was reading. He loved everything from Sci-fi to Dean Koontz to the Classics. One of his favorites as a young child was "Where the Red Fern Grows," and more recent was "Watchers." He got really good grades in every subject and was liked and respected by all his teachers and counselors all through his school years.

One thing that I miss the most about Christopher is his quick and charming wit and his wonderful sense of humor. His favorite holiday was Halloween, and believe me, he and his brother Peter made the most of it! His second, was Christmas. We had a lot of family traditions. Making cookies, cutting down our Christmas tree, caroling and reading "The Polar Express" on Christmas Eve, with George and me jingling sleigh bells after they had gone to bed. It was always so much fun, even as the boys got older!

We also loved to travel. We took the boys to Japan several years ago. If any of you start craving sushi, that's from Chris! He picked up on the language right away and did some minor translating for all of us. He was only ten years old! We also took a lot of ski vacations, both in the U.S. and Canada. Chris started skiing at age five, so by age fifteen, before the accident, he was a very accomplished and tremendous skier.

Christopher enjoyed and appreciated nature. He would describe to us the beauty he saw in the sky and walking in the quietness of the snow. He was very expressive for his age.

I hope you enjoyed meeting Christopher. We miss him terribly, but we know he totally approved of our choice to donate. He was very giving and caring. We wish you all the best of health and happiness.

With caring regards and in loving memory of Christopher,

George, Joni, and Peter

In addition to the letter for all the recipients of Christopher's organs, the Kuhlmans sent this letter to me.

Dearest Heart Recipient,

Thank you so much for the letters from all of you, and thank you most recently for your card. That was so thoughtful to remember us on this first anniversary. We all really appreciated it. It was a very difficult couple of weeks. Actually, this past year has been pretty awful. But even after his death we have learned a lot from him.

He was a great young man. I don't know if you know any details of his death. He was walking home and was hit by a car. It all happened so fast. Christopher didn't suffer; we were told he didn't feel any pain or have time to be afraid.

We would like to meet you and your family sometime! We want you to know that we're really happy for you. And very, very proud of how well you did at the Transplant Olympics. Christopher loved to swim!

You have a very kind, thoughtful, and strong heart!!

With fond regards,

George, Joni and Peter

About a year after Christopher died, his younger brother, Peter, wrote him this letter. It was included in a display about transplants in the Hall of Life at the Museum of Nature and Science in Denver.

You know, Chris, I think about a lot of things, especially about when you were here. You always gave me so much encouragement. One thing I didn't think of was that you might die unexpectedly. I'm doing all kinds of things now, working, skateboarding, and snowboarding. I wish you were here.

I remember you saying that you always wanted to help people. You died, so it's kind of hard now, but you did help so many people, because we made the decision to donate your organs and tissues. You helped a lot of people and I'm very proud of you for that. In fact, once I get my driver's license, I'm going to sign the back of it so that I can be a donor.

Sometimes kids will ask me, why would you want to donate your brother's organs and tissues? I tell them that not only would my brother want us to do that exact thing, but also it was the right thing to do.

I'll always love you,

Peter

Christopher wrote this poem when he was twelve, three years before he died.

Sit and reminisce the days of old
Remember the
Lilac Springs, we were its bees, it was our hive
And how we enjoyed them, as they enjoyed us
Swimming and splashing like fish
Without a clue of what the future had in store
Now wish
Hope
Return just once
No
It can never be the same
It can only happen
In dream land
BUT WAIT!
There is yet a way to return
Forever
Endless Sleep
A forever dream land
But is it worth it
What has been achieved?
Nothing
It is a worthless triumph to some
But to me...

Appendix 2

Laura's Report of Our First Meeting with the Kuhlmans

Laura Roiger's letter about Christopher's last night appeared earlier in this book. She was also there the day we met the Kuhlmans. This is her report:

There are experiences in life that stick with you, never to be forgotten. One such experience for me was February 14, 1999, when I witnessed two families meet for the first time. Although the families had never met one another before, I believe they knew each other more intimately than had they been life-long acquaintances. Valentine's Day this year would take on a new meaning for me and never be the same again.

It's almost noon and I'm standing with reporters and others whose lives have intersected because of Christopher and Gaea. I don't know if I'm shaking from the cool air or because

I'm nervous and excited to witness what seems like a very holy union.

I see Gaea and her family for the first time and, because I'm a nurse, do a quick visual exam of Gaea and notice how healthy and vibrant she looks. She exudes a sense of warmth and her smile cannot be erased, although I sense some nervousness.

As Joni, George, and Peter walk towards Gaea and her family, Joni picks up her pace, asks if she could listen to Christopher's heart beat, and places her ear to Gaea's chest. A union of two women—one with a broken heart and the other with a heart of gratitude for the life given to her.

The work I do as an ICU nurse who takes care of many who die is often difficult and emotionally draining, but the experience of witnessing this meeting affirms that what I do is important and in many ways life-giving.

Every Valentine's Day I remember what I experienced when the Kuhlmans and Shaws met, and I am reminded of what it really means to give your heart to someone. Every time I see Gaea, I feel a warm sense of gratitude to Christopher's family for the life they gave to her, that allowed her to touch so many lives since receiving his heart.

At the same time, I continue to be aware of the painful loss these wonderful people will forever carry because Christopher's life was so short. I pray the hole they feel in their hearts is filled with some peace knowing that in his death, Christopher made a big difference in the lives of so many people.

Appendix 3

Coach Liz's Report

My coach sent this report to World T.E.A.M./The Greg LeMond Grant Program. It resulted in my receiving a small grant for the 2003 World Games in France.

A lifeguard's main job is the safety of patrons in the water. In early1998 when a frail, petite woman entered the pool on my shift, my attention focused on this woman attempting to swim laps. Her swimming was a slow paddle and I did not think she was going to make it to the far side of the pool. I was ready to rescue. She finally made it and looked at me with a huge smile, gripped the side of the pool and catching her breath, then began to swim back. Again I was ready to rescue this determined swimmer. I was relieved when she finished her lap and climbed out of the pool with the biggest smile, not the panicked look of a distressed swimmer.

She introduced herself and thanked me for keeping an eagle's eye on her as she swam, and she confided that she wasn't sure she was going to make it. I was instantly amazed at this woman's determination when she said she would be back tomorrow to swim. Gaea Shaw did come back the next day. That is when I learned about her remarkable life.

Gaea had just received a heart transplant. Needing to exercise, she felt a spirit guiding her to the water. She was never a swimmer but was willing to learn and asked me for lessons. We started with the basics: reach, pull, kick, and breathe. She enjoyed learning and I noticed how easy it was for her to process what I taught her. It seemed like she had two coaches encouraging her because she learned so quickly.

Because of Gaea's new life, new heart, she wanted to take advantage of everything life had to offer, and that included competing in the 1998 U.S. Transplant Games that were being held in Columbus, Ohio. I went from being a teacher to coach the very next day. Gaea did not have a competitive attitude at first. Her main goal was just to be able to look good when she swam and to be able to at least finish in all her events. It quickly became apparent to me that her hard work in the pool was going to reward her at the games, so I encouraged her to swim faster, and each timed practice swim was better then the last. Gaea certainly felt the spirit within move her through the water during the games because she won two gold medals and one silver medal! I was very proud of her and amazed at her "go for it" attitude.

Gaea's love for the sport of swimming kept growing and, in addition to our coaching sessions, Gaea joined a master's swim team. Her dedication to swimming was bewildering to me, the lifeguard who was ready to rescue that petite, frail lady who could barely swim just months earlier.

Next, the 2000 Transplant Games were on the horizon and Gaea was a driving force behind our local transplant group, Team Rocky Mountain. She rallied extraordinary people who had various transplants and convinced them that they, too, could learn to swim, compete, and win. What a motivator! I soon was coaching six swimmers. Her enthusiasm and encouragement toward her teammates made my job easy. Everyone really learned to swim well, and the personal best goals that Gaea set for herself became the benchmark for the team, with all the swimmers soon wanting to be just like Gaea. Our entire team did great at the games, and Gaea won three silver medals in her events. Although the medals were not gold I truly believe she felt she did win the biggest, brightest gold medal there ever will be when she received her new heart.

Gaea's donor heart came from a teenage boy who was passionate about water and music. Gaea met his family in 1999, and his mother and brother attended the games in 2000. Gaea presented them with the medals she won, thanking them for their gift of life. His heart may be beating in Gaea's body but his soul and love for swimming helped teach this special lady how to enjoy everything the water has to offer. Gaea's zest for living life to the fullest made her the athlete she has become.

In 2001 Gaea competed at the International Games in Kobe, Japan, and came home with a gold medal. She was very excited to compete abroad and have the opportunity to meet other transplant athletes. Her ambassador-like personality drew people toward her. She genuinely supported her competitors in all their events and has made many friends throughout the world.

Since I met Gaea she has been to six competitions and has won medals each time. She is an athlete in mind, body, spirit, and soul. I have known this wonderful lady for seven years and know how hard she works to be able to go to these events. Each time Gaea attends the games, the experience of meeting, competing, and honoring transplant and donor families makes it worth every cent spent getting there. Anyone in the stands on opening night would feel the wonderful energy that all the athletes give to living, not just to competing.

Gaea's health is great and her heart is that of a fifteen-year-old swimmer whose soul belongs in the water. She has made such great use of her new life, achieved many goals and spread her goodwill to so many people. She who I thought at first needed rescuing, in fact rescued many people, including her donor family, by showing them how life does go on. To transplant recipients waiting for organs she proves that there is hope for a better life. In her own way, Gaea rescued herself by enjoying every second, living life to its fullest with everything she does, and she does it well. She shares with everyone the passion of competition and the honor that goes hand in hand with being an athlete.

Appendix 4

In Lieu of Flowers, Consider Donation

The statistics are staggering. As of this writing there are over 87,000 people in the U.S. waiting for a transplant. Only a small percentage of them will be lucky enough to get one. Every day thirteen new patients are added to the transplant waiting list. And every day seventeen people die waiting for an organ.

About half the states have donor registries, which means that people can declare in advance their decision to be a donor. In some states, such as Colorado, if a person's name is on the registry, this is the permission needed for organ donation and the family's consent is neither needed nor asked for. They are informed of the person's decision to be an organ donor, and the people from the organ procurement agency offer support and spend time helping the family understand what that means. In other states the donor registry is only an indication of the persons wishes, and the family's consent is still needed to proceed. Letting your family know you want to be a donor will help them with this process and increase the possibility of your wishes being honored.

I was lucky to get my heart and that luck is bothersome. Why should luck play a part in a person's ability to get a life-saving transplant? The year I received my new heart, eight hundred people died in the U. S. because a heart didn't come in time.

Look at some of the websites about organ donation. All of them educate. Some offer specific help for donor families and recipients. Become inspired. If you haven't registered to become a donor, let the facts dispel some long-held myths. You have the opportunity to save someone's life. You can become someone's hero.

I thank my donor every day. I'm looking at Christopher's picture right now.

http://www.americantransplant.org
American Transplant Association, Inc.

980 N. Michigan Ave.

Suite 1400-#1402

Chicago, IL 60611

800-494-4527

Ask for their book, "A Patient's Guide to Transplantation." It has extensive appendices on financial assistance, medications, religious views on organ donation, and support resources.

http://www.donoralliance.org/
Donor Alliance is a non-profit organization that facilitates donation and recovery of organs and tissues in Colorado and Wyoming. Check out the excellent resources link for a comprehensive list of donation-related websites.

http://www.donor-awareness.org
The Donor Awareness Council is dedicated to increasing organ and tissue donation through education and awareness in Wyoming and Colorado. The stories and the discussion of myths and religion are global issues, not related to locale. Worth looking at.

http://www.kidney.org/
National Kidney Foundation

30 E. 33rd Street

New York, NY 10016

(800)622-9010

For information on kidney disease, organ donation, transplantation, and the National Kidney Foundation's Olympic-style U.S. Transplant Games.

http://organtransplants.org
Learn about all aspects of the journey, with stories of donor families and transplant recipients. Hear some of the stories on your computer speakers.

http://www.donatelife.net, http://www.donevida.org (Spanish)
The Coalition on Donation is a national organization founded by the transplant community to educate the public about organ and tissue donation. A U.S. map on the website links to state specific donor information.

http://www.transplantbuddies.org/
Personal stories about the transplant journey; on-line mentors for every type of transplant.

http://www.transweb.org/
TransWeb: All About Transplantation and Donation is a nonprofit educational web site serving the world transplant community. Based at the University of Michigan, TransWeb features news and events, real people's experiences, the top ten myths about donation, a donation quiz, and a large collection of questions and answers, as well as a reference area with everything from articles to videos. For adults and teens, TransWeb features "Give Life: The Transplant Journey," a multimedia trip through the donation and transplantation process.

Appendix 5

How to Create a Phone Tree

By planning ahead and creating a phone tree, you can contact many people in just a few minutes. In our situation, we made only three calls. From there, eighty people were contacted. We found this invaluable for all the stages of the journey—when I learned that there was a heart for me, when I went into surgery, when I came out of surgery, and when I needed support once I came home. Here's how we did it.

We made a list of everyone we wanted to contact.

We grouped them first by importance for immediate support and, after that, by area code.

Each person on the tree had only three to five people to call, and most of the calls were within their area code, so there was a minimum of long distance calling.

A copy of the phone tree was sent to everyone. If anyone didn't want to make calls, they were asked to inform me immediately so I could substitute someone else.

This is the letter we sent with the phone tree:

Phone Tree for Gaea

In an effort to get the word out to many people quickly that I'm in the hospital, about my progress, etc., I've created this phone tree.

- *If you have a group of people to call and don't want that responsibility, please let me know immediately so I can find someone else to do it.*

- *For obvious reasons, please keep this list in a safe place.*

- *If you have a group to call and you get someone's voice mail, ask them to return your call. That way you'll know everyone on your list has gotten the news.*

- *If you find that someone on your list is out of town or otherwise completely unreachable, please make their phone calls for them if they have a group to call.*

Gaea's Phone Tree

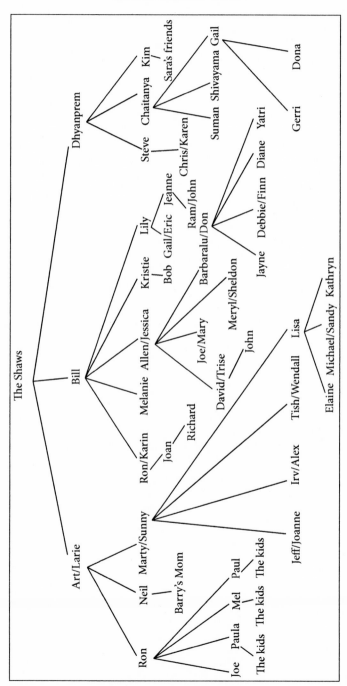

Notes

Printed in the United States
27255LVS00001B/232-705